PRACTICAL
DIABETES CARE
For Healthcare Professionals

PRACTICAL
DIABETES CARE
For Healthcare Professionals

Second Edition

Sora Ludwig, MD, FRCPC
Professor, Endocrinology and Metabolism,
Faculty of Health Sciences,
Max Rady College of Medicine,
University of Manitoba, Winnipeg, Canada

ELSEVIER

Elsevier
Radarweg 29, PO Box 211, 1000 AE Amsterdam, Netherlands
The Boulevard, Langford Lane, Kidlington, Oxford OX5 1GB, United Kingdom
50 Hampshire Street, 5th Floor, Cambridge, MA 02139, United States

Library of Congress Cataloging-in-Publication Data
A catalog record for this book is available from the Library of Congress

British Library Cataloguing-in-Publication Data
A catalogue record for this book is available from the British Library

ISBN: 978-0-12-820082-7

For information on all Elsevier publications visit our website
at https://www.elsevier.com/books-and-journals

Publisher: Stacy Masucci
Acquisitions Editor: Ana Claudia Garcia
Editorial Project Manager: Kristi Anderson
Production Project Manager: Swapna Srinivasan
Cover Designer: Miles Hitchen

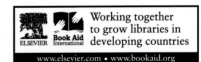
Working together
to grow libraries in
developing countries

www.elsevier.com • www.bookaid.org

Typeset by TNQ Technologies

CONTENTS

AUTHOR ACKNOWLEDGMENTS

I would like to acknowledge the hard work of all the professional volunteers who have contributed to the *Diabetes Canada Clinical Practice Guidelines for the Prevention and Management of Diabetes in Canada* over the years, including myself. Their combined efforts have helped me in writing this handbook. I would also like to acknowledge Elsevier and Diabetes Canada for granting permission to use certain figures throughout this handbook.

I would also like to acknowledge Dr. John Embil for contributing his expertise to the Neuropathy section of the "Chronic Complications of Diabetes: Assessment and Management" chapter.

I would also like to acknowledge the effort of Fiona Hendry, the medical editor who worked diligently alongside me throughout this process.

INTRODUCTION

I have been a practicing endocrinologist for more than 30 years. As with most endocrinologists, approximately 75% of my practice is diabetes related. I have thoroughly enjoyed every minute of my practice and hope to continue this job for years to come. As a professor of medicine and full-time faculty member at the University of Manitoba, I have spent considerable time teaching medical students, physicians in postgraduate training programs, family physicians in practice, and many allied healthcare professionals, including Certified Diabetes Educators, nurse practitioners, physician assistants, nurses, dietitians, pharmacists, social workers, and community health workers. Along the way, I have developed the ability to translate evidence-based clinical practice guidelines into the reality of daily clinical practice in diabetes.

I wanted to share my experienced-based approaches to diabetes. In 2013, I wrote the first edition of *Practical Diabetes Care for Healthcare Professionals*. This handbook was targeted to all healthcare professionals involved in diabetes care. Since these groups are, for the most part, involved in the care of people with type 2 (T2) diabetes, the first edition of this handbook was limited to a discussion of T2 diabetes.

In this edition, I have expanded the discussion to include many aspects of type 1 (T1) diabetes as well as aspects of T2 diabetes not covered in the first edition. Diabetic ketoacidosis (DKA), an acute complication most often associated with T1 diabetes, is discussed; the acute T2 diabetes complication of hyperglycemic hyperosmolar nonketotic (HHNK) state is also addressed. Also, there is more information about hypoglycemia, long-term complications, and the many pharmacologic and technologic developments that have occurred in diabetes management. Certainly, with the many recent advances in diabetes care, particularly in T2 diabetes, it is time for the now internationally expanded edition of *Practical Diabetes Care for Healthcare Professionals*.

Diabetes primer
Type 1 diabetes

T1 diabetes is an autoimmune disease that affects the insulin-producing beta islet cells of the pancreas, resulting in an absolute deficiency of pancreatic insulin secretion. Therefore people with T1 diabetes, in the absence of insulin, are at risk for the acute symptoms of hyperglycemia (e.g., polydipsia, polyuria, blurred vision, unexplained weight loss) and eventual metabolic

Practical Diabetes Care for Healthcare Professionals
ISBN 978-0-12-820082-7
https://doi.org/10.1016/B978-0-12-820082-7.00001-4

decompensation evolving into DKA. Overall, people with T1 diabetes require insulin from the time of diagnosis.

People with T1 diabetes are managed quite differently from those with T2 diabetes. They may experience more labile blood glucose control and are best managed with a team approach, usually referred to as the diabetes healthcare (DHC) team, with care shared among the endocrinologist, primary care provider, and professional diabetes educators who are experienced in the care of T1 diabetes.

Type 2 diabetes

T2 diabetes has a much different pathophysiology than T1 diabetes. It is associated with varying degrees of insulin resistance in insulin's target tissues of the liver, skeletal muscle, and adipose tissue, as well as pancreatic insulin secretion deficiency. In essence, people with T2 diabetes still have sufficient insulin so they are less prone to acute metabolic decompensation and DKA. However, they may be prone to another acute complication, HHNK state. People with T2 diabetes often respond to a combination of oral and/or injectable antihyperglycemic medications, including insulin.

T2 diabetes is on the rise not only in Canada but also around the world. With this increased prevalence, it would be frankly impossible for specialist teams to care for everyone with diabetes, particularly T2 diabetes. Accordingly, evidence-based clinical practice guidelines have been developed by many recognized diabetes organizations with the purpose of disseminating diabetes management knowledge and skills from specialists into the hands of primary care practitioners. Unfortunately, this approach often does not work. By virtue of being evidence-based, clinical guidelines are broad-based; therefore, unfortunately, they are not practical. They require logical interpretation if they are to be used appropriately and widely. It is the objective of this handbook to provide the practical aspect to translate guideline dissemination into daily implementation.

It is important to remember that diabetes care and management is chronic and lifelong. It is multifaceted, affecting a person's daily life, family, and workplace. Beyond the usual physical health impact, diabetes may carry a significant psychological and emotional burden. Successful care means whole (person) care, which can be daunting for an individual healthcare provider. Team care—such as a DHC team—can make a significant difference. Teams can be on-site, off-site, virtual, fluid in their composition and changing as the needs of the person with diabetes change. The DHC team care approach to T2 diabetes is growing as the population with diabetes grows and the need for care increases.

ORGANIZATION OF DIABETES CARE

Abstract

Diabetes is primarily self-managed. People with diabetes must commit themselves to a daily balance of lifestyle choices with respect to food intake and physical activity, in association with frequent monitoring of blood glucose levels and the use of medications (i.e., antihyperglycemic agents, insulin, or both). The concept of the diabetes healthcare (DHC) team, where the person with diabetes is at the center surrounded by a core of healthcare professionals, is well recognized as providing the most successful long-term care for diabetes. There have also been increasing technologic advances in office practice organization that make this system more efficient. However, it is recognized that living well with diabetes can be stressful and this is where an expanded DHC team can provide the necessary emotional and psychologic support as well.

Keywords: Certified diabetes educator; Diabetes healthcare team; Living with diabetes; Reminder and recall systems; Shared care.

Practical Diabetes Care for Healthcare Professionals
ISBN 978-0-12-820082-7
https://doi.org/10.1016/B978-0-12-820082-7.00002-6

The diabetes healthcare team

Diabetes is primarily self-managed. People with diabetes must commit themselves to a daily lifestyle regimen with respect to food intake and physical activity, often in association with medications (i.e., antihyperglycemic agents, insulin, or both). These demands of daily life may be difficult to accomplish alone, both for the person with diabetes trying to cope and for the primary care provider who is trying to help them manage their diabetes. Expertise and experience in understanding diabetes and its management are required, including dietary counseling, the effect of exercise, the often unrecognized effect of emotional stress, self-monitoring of blood glucose (SMBG) levels, insulin administration, interpreting blood glucose patterns, and being aware of the ever-evolving diabetes technologies.

Diabetes was one of the first medical specialties to adopt a team approach to patient care, and the concept of the diabetes healthcare (DHC) team is now well accepted in clinical practice. The goal of the DHC team is to provide the person with diabetes with the skills to successfully self-manage their diabetes. Although this is a tall order, and can take months or years to achieve, it has proven successful in real-world clinical care settings.

At the center of the DHC team is the person with diabetes. Most often, the core team consists of an endocrinologist and/or a primary care provider and diabetes educators—a nurse and a dietitian—preferably Certified Diabetes Educators (CDEs), i.e., individuals who have obtained a standardized certification in diabetes education. Other members who may contribute to the team include a pharmacist, an optometrist and/or ophthalmologist or retinal specialist, a podiatrist, a kinesiologist, a dentist and/or a dental hygienist, and a mental health worker (i.e., psychiatrist, psychologist, or social worker), as well as trained peer supports.

Shared care

Successful diabetes management occurs when the DHC team shares the care with the primary care provider. It cannot be overstated that the central team member is the person with diabetes, followed closely by the primary support network of family and friends.

Importantly, research has demonstrated that people with type 1 (T1) diabetes have better outcomes working within a shared care model with a DHC team that includes an endocrinologist and CDEs. This is related to the level of complexity that can often arise in the management of T1 diabetes. Advanced DHC teams, i.e., those that include CDEs, can provide additional support in managing complex diabetes medication regimens, insulin pumps, continuous glucose monitoring systems, specific diabetes problem-solving, and individualized case management. They can also help those with diabetes cope with the day-to-day stress of juggling nutritional intake, physical activity, and medication regimens.

People with type 2 (T2) diabetes with complex management requirements (e.g., secondary to diabetes-related complications) may also benefit from interaction with a DHC team that includes CDEs.

For those people with less complex T2 diabetes the DHC team may look different, with a primary care provider—rather than an endocrinologist—and the involvement of community-based diabetes educators. Many local healthcare jurisdictions have community-based diabetes education resource centers that provide patient education and counseling regarding nutrition, physical activity, SMBG instruction, and insulin administration. When necessary, the DHC team can expand to include other healthcare providers and community service professionals and providers.

Endocrinologists/diabetes specialists may take on roles beyond the customary consultant role; indeed, they may act as mentors, educators, and facilitators of shared-care and/or case management approaches with a primary care provider. The traditional role of the specialist consultant is evolving as team-based care in many clinical areas is becoming more common.

Reminder and recall systems
Clinical organizational practices that have been shown to improve the care of people with diabetes include reminder and recall systems for the physician, the DHC team, and the person with diabetes. These systems render the regular monitoring of diabetes and its complications an automatic function. Depending on the individual clinic situation, reminder and recall systems are increasingly centralized through electronic scheduling systems. Electronic medical records (EMRs) are also very common now. Depending on the function of an EMR, ongoing flow sheets of key laboratory results can be generated, allowing the DHC team to review changing values over time, e.g., levels of glycated hemoglobin (A1C). Abnormal laboratory results can be flagged and even linked to evidence-based clinical practice guidelines that provide management recommendations. Such systems can facilitate individual diabetes case management and specific problem-solving by DHC team members.

For those healthcare professionals who are not using electronic systems, various paper tools can still prove useful. Diabetes care plans, flow sheets, and other similar charts and forms can be used to maintain updated patient profiles and chronicle any complications by tracking clinical and laboratory data.

Living with diabetes

It has been said that one can never take a holiday from their diabetes. Truer words were never spoken! There is no break or remission from diabetes. Blood glucose levels continue to fluctuate with food intake, activity, and physical or emotional stress. Individuals must constantly balance the nuances of daily life with their medications, all the while attempting to maintain optimal target blood glucose levels as advised by their DHC team. It is a long-term game plan to prevent or delay the development or progression of chronic diabetes complications.

At the time of diagnosis, individual reactions vary. With an acute presentation of either T1 or T2 diabetes, the initial reaction may be one of disbelief, followed quickly by a form of reactive depression and sometimes anger. Other times, the emotional reaction surfaces days or weeks later as the reality of the diagnosis sinks in. Recognizing and providing support for these reactions is crucial to the future ability of the person to manage and cope with their diabetes.

It can be very helpful if a person's initial introduction to diabetes and all it entails is a positive one. Staying positive in the face of this often-unexpected diagnosis can be very difficult for the individual. This is where the initial interaction with the DHC team can be very useful. The team can provide that all-important initial and ongoing support as well as expert knowledge. At times, it can be very helpful to have access to a mental health counselor, a psychologist, or even a psychiatrist as an adjunct to the core DHC team. For some people with diabetes, access to experienced peer support can also prove beneficial.

The expectation of lifelong maintenance of those key diabetes targets for blood glucose levels and targets to reduce the risk of complications (e.g., blood pressure, cholesterol) can take its toll on a person. The daily burden of diabetes management is added to the daily burden of life, school, job, work, and family commitments and responsibilities. Often, with other more pressing issues at hand, diabetes may drop to the bottom of a person's priority list, only to be thought of once other issues have resolved.

I find that diabetes can take on this "roller-coaster" pattern in many individuals. It helps to acknowledge that real-life stresses can stand in the way of optimal diabetes management and also that those roller-coaster patterns of diabetes self-management are going to occur but hopefully will improve with time. The reality of barriers to successful self-management must be recognized and the person supported before the diabetes can again be addressed.

I like to think that a successful diabetes self-manager is the person who "runs" their diabetes and does not let diabetes "run" them. It is incumbent on the wider DHC team to help the person develop coping skills that will help them manage their diabetes over the long term. It is also important to realize that this is indeed a tall order and that there are no quick fixes for diabetes self-management.

DIABETES CARE IN THE OFFICE

Abstract

Type 1 and type 2 diabetes are very different entities. The differences in how they present to the healthcare system and how they differ in pathogenesis are discussed in this chapter. Risk factors for the development of diabetes and screening for diabetes are also reviewed. A discussion about the impact of prediabetes and metabolic syndrome of insulin resistance is also included. Much of this chapter is devoted to detailing the office clinical assessment of the person newly diagnosed with diabetes, including pertinent points regarding clinical history, physical examination, and laboratory investigations. This information is presented in a practical checklist form, for the most part.

Keywords: Clinical checklists; Metabolic syndrome of insulin resistance; Prediabetes; Type 1 diabetes; Type 2 diabetes.

Practical Diabetes Care for Healthcare Professionals
ISBN 978-0-12-820082-7
https://doi.org/10.1016/B978-0-12-820082-7.00003-8

Introduction

Diabetes care comprises a significant amount of routine office practice for the primary care provider. As with all chronic conditions, diabetes takes *time*. Also, with recognition of the complications associated with diabetes, it is no longer sufficient to simply review blood glucose levels with patients. A complete assessment of people with diabetes must also include a review of diabetes medications and other medication regimens, glycemic control, nutritional intake, physical activity, and a discussion about stress and its detrimental effect on blood glucose control. Also, importantly, an assessment for any possible long-term micro- and macrovascular complications must be completed. All these components play a role in successful diabetes management.

Awareness of diabetes and its growing impact is the first step in practice. With the prevalence of diabetes increasing at an astounding rate, it is important to recognize the risk factors for diabetes and screen appropriately.

Type 1 versus type 2 diabetes

As is well known, type 1 (T1) diabetes is a chronic condition whereby the pancreatic islet cells are destroyed through an autoimmune process. Certain demographics characterize T1 diabetes: it occurs more commonly in children and adolescents but can also be seen in older adults. T1 diabetes is characterized by complete insulin deficiency, necessitating prompt recognition and treatment with insulin. In type 2 (T2) diabetes, there is a variable degree of insulin resistance as well as insulin deficiency. Depending on the individual, management may include a combination of oral and/or parenteral antihyperglycemic medications and/or insulin.

Research has shown that the management of T1 diabetes is best accomplished through a shared care model with an endocrinologist, an experienced diabetes healthcare (DHC) team, and a primary care provider. T2 diabetes can often be managed successfully with a primary care provider and a community-based DHC team.

The information that follows applies generally to those with either T1 or T2 diabetes; however, at times the information is centered on T2 diabetes, as it is managed most often in the primary care setting.

Diabetes screening

It is not recommended that screening for T1 diabetes be conducted routinely. Although there is an increased genetic risk in families with T1 diabetes, regular screening of nonaffected family members is not advised. Awareness of presenting symptoms is helpful to recognize possible T1 diabetes early in its onset.

As T2 diabetes may be asymptomatic, there may be significant lag time between true onset and diagnosis of the condition. Accordingly, recognition of the potential risk factors and active screening for T2 diabetes is key.

Risk factors for T2 diabetes include the following:

- Age ≥40 years
- First-degree relative with T2 diabetes
- Member of a high-risk ethnic group: Indigenous, Hispanic, Asian, South Asian, or African descent
- Associated conditions of insulin resistance, including impaired glucose tolerance (IGT), impaired fasting glucose (IFG), prediabetes, polycystic ovarian syndrome, gestational diabetes mellitus, acanthosis nigricans, or metabolic syndrome of insulin resistance
- The presence of cardiovascular risk factors, such as hypertension, abdominal obesity, or obstructive sleep apnea
- The presence of psychiatric disorders, including schizophrenia, bipolar disease, depression, and/or the use of atypical antipsychotic medications
- The use of medications known to be associated with diabetes, such as glucocorticoids and highly active antiretroviral therapy

Diagnosis of diabetes

The diagnosis of diabetes is straightforward, and there are a number of diagnostic methods:

- *Random plasma glucose ≥11.1 mmol/L* in the presence of typical symptoms, including polydipsia, polyuria, blurred vision, extreme fatigue, or unintended weight loss.
- *Fasting plasma glucose (FPG) ≥7.0 mmol/L* in the absence of typical symptoms (where fasting means no caloric intake for at least 8 hours).
- *Glycated hemoglobin (A1C) >6.5%* is another valid diagnostic test for diabetes. It is important to remember, however, that some factors, such as iron deficiency, may affect A1C values.
- The gold-standard test remains *a 2 hour plasma glucose ≥11.1 mmol/L in a 75-g oral glucose tolerance test (OGTT).*

Normally, the diagnostic test for diabetes should be confirmed on another day, *but a delay of treatment should not occur in those persons who are symptomatic, showing signs of metabolic decompensation (i.e., significant hyperglycemia or unexpected weight loss), or suspected to have T1 diabetes.* Table 3.1 summarizes the diagnostic criteria for diabetes.

Diagnostic criteria for diabetes

FPG ≥7.0 mmol/L
or
A1C ≥6.5% (in adults)
or
2-hour PG in a 75 g OGTT ≥11.1 mmol/L
or
Random PG ≥11.1 mmol/L

2-hour PG, 2 hour plasma glucose; *A1C*, glycated hemoglobin; *FPG*, fasting plasma glucose; *OGTT*, oral glucose tolerance test; *PG*, plasma glucose.

Diagnosis of prediabetes

Prediabetes defines an earlier stage of glucose intolerance, identified as either IGT or IFG. A1C values of 6.0%–6.4% are also diagnostic indicators for prediabetes.

However, some individuals with lower blood glucose levels may still be at increased risk for diabetes. Accordingly, anyone with an FPG of 6.1–6.9 mmol/L or an A1C of 5.5%–5.9%, in the presence of diabetes risk factors, should be screened with a 75-g OGTT. Besides being at greater risk from converting to T2 diabetes, prediabetes, particularly IGT, confers a separate increased risk for the development of cardiovascular disease (CVD). Thus there is value in recognizing prediabetes. Table 3.2 summarizes the diagnostic criteria for prediabetes.

TABLE 3.2

Diagnosis of prediabetes

Test	Result	Prediabetes category
FPG (mmol/L)	6.1–6.9	IFG
2-hour PG in a 75-g OGTT (mmol/L)	7.8–11.0	IGT
A1C (%)	6.0–6.4	Prediabetes

2-hour PG, 2 hour plasma glucose; *A1C*, glycated hemoglobin; *FPG*, fasting plasma glucose; *IFG*, impaired fasting glucose; *IGT*, impaired glucose tolerance; *OGTT*, oral glucose tolerance test.

Management of prediabetes

Research has demonstrated overwhelmingly that lifestyle changes (i.e., healthy eating and increased physical activity) can delay or prevent the conversion of prediabetes to T2 diabetes. The challenge is that these changes must be consistent and maintained over time. Pharmacologic therapy for these patients (e.g., an insulin sensitizer such as metformin) can be considered. However, it may be difficult for patients to commit to long-term pharmacologic therapy for a condition that they do not necessarily consider an adverse medical condition. Working diligently with a nonpharmacologic approach is generally deemed to be the most acceptable choice for patients. As prediabetes confers a separate risk for CVD, it is important to screen and propose a strategy for any other modifiable CVD risk factors, including smoking, hypertension, and dyslipidemia.

Diagnosis of metabolic syndrome of insulin resistance

Metabolic syndrome of insulin resistance (i.e., metabolic syndrome) refers to a constellation of conditions that confer a high risk of CVD in an individual. These conditions include prediabetes, diabetes, hypertension, dyslipidemia, and abdominal obesity, most of which can be modified. Table 3.3 lists the clinical characteristics for diagnosing metabolic syndrome.

TABLE 3.3

Clinical characteristics for diagnosing metabolic syndrome

Risk factor	Threshold value	
	Men	Women
Elevated waist circumference (cm)		
Canada, United States	≥102	≥88
Europid, Middle Eastern, sub-Saharan African, Mediterranean	≥94	≥80
Asian, Japanese, South and Central American	≥90	≥80
TG (mmol/L)	≥1.7	
HDL-C (mmol/L)		
Men	<1.0	
Women	<1.3	

Continued

TABLE 3.3

Clinical characteristics for diagnosing metabolic
syndrome—cont'd

Risk factor	Threshold value	
	Men	Women
BP (mm Hg)	≥130/85	
FPG (mmol/L)	≥5.6	

BP, blood pressure; *FPG*, fasting plasma glucose; *HDL-C*, high-density lipoprotein cholesterol;
TG, triglyceride.

Implications for metabolic syndrome are as follows:
- Recognition
- Insulin resistance as the key characteristic; therefore, the need to screen for prediabetes/T2 diabetes
- Multipronged management approach for the modifiable components

Diabetes: clinical assessment

Although the clinical assessment described here can pertain to newly diagnosed T1 or T2 diabetes, it may have greater relevance for T2 diabetes because of the recognized lag time between onset and diagnosis. It is particularly important to assess for the presence of chronic complications at the time of diagnosis, as the time of true onset of diabetes often predates the time of diagnosis; thus, chronic complications may already be present.

For the person newly diagnosed with diabetes, a complete clinical assessment is necessary. This should include assessment of acute complications, including symptoms of hyperglycemia, as well as the presence of any chronic microvascular complications (e.g., retinopathy, neuropathy, nephropathy) and macrovascular complications (e.g., CVD, peripheral or cerebral vascular disease).

For the person with known diabetes, initial evaluation should include the abovementioned, as well as information-gathering regarding past and current diabetes medications (including medications for diabetes-related complications), previous diabetes education experience, and assessment of diabetes knowledge.

Checklist for diabetes assessment

- **Current status**
  - Symptoms of hyperglycemia
    - Polydipsia
    - Polyuria
    - Blurred vision
    - Skin, vaginal, or urinary tract infection
    - Unexpected weight loss

- **Diabetes assessment**
  - Current diabetes medications
  - Previous diabetes education knowledge and skills, including self-monitoring of blood glucose (SMBG), insulin administration, and dosage adjustment
  - Nutritional intake, including meal and snack patterns, and food choices
  - Weight history
  - Physical activity
  - Family history of diabetes
  - Social determinants of health, including family or caregiver supports, work type, financial issues, and health beliefs

- **Diabetes complication assessment**
  - Medications for diabetes-related complications
  - Retinopathy
    - Date of last retinal assessment
    - Blurred vision or other visual disturbances
  - Neuropathy
    - Diffuse symmetric polyneuropathy
    - Focal mononeuropathies
    - Autonomic neuropathies: hypoglycemia unawareness, gastrointestinal, genital/urinary (including erectile dysfunction), cardiovascular (postural hypotension)
  - Nephropathy
    - Hypertension
  - CVD, peripheral or cerebral vascular disease
    - Dyslipidemia
    - Angina, myocardial infarction
    - Transient ischemic attack, cerebral vascular accident
    - Claudication, foot ulcers

- **General assessment**
  - Additional health problems, including mental health issues
    - T1 diabetes can be associated with other autoimmune conditions, including thyroid, celiac disease, and rheumatologic disorders
  - Other medications, including nonprescription medications
  - Allergies
  - Smoking, alcohol, and recreational drug history

- **Physical examination**
  - General
    - Weight, body mass index, and waist circumference
    - Blood pressure
  - Systems (assessing for complications)
    - Eye
      - Cataracts
      - Fundoscopic examination (does not replace retinal assessment through dilated pupils by an experienced examiner)
    - Oral: teeth and gums
    - Thyroid (thyroid disorders are common; however, there is no specific relationship to T2 diabetes but a definite association in autoimmune T1 diabetes)
    - Foot examination
      - Screening for vascular integrity
        - ✔ Color
        - ✔ Skin and nail condition
        - ✔ Peripheral pulses
      - Screening for peripheral neuropathy
        - ✔ 10-g Semmes-Weinstein monofilament test (see Chronic Complications of Diabetes chapter for the technique)
        - ✔ Presence of vibration sense or proprioception
        - ✔ Presence of infection or ulceration
        - ✔ Presence of ankle reflexes

- **Investigations**
  - Glycemic control
    - Glycated hemoglobin (A1C)
    - Review of SMBG or continuous glucose monitoring records

- Complications assessment
  - Complete blood count
  - Electrolytes
  - Liver function
  - Renal function
    - Urine albumin/creatinine ratio (uACR)
    - Serum creatinine levels
    - Estimated glomerular filtration rate (eGFR)
  - Lipid profile
  - Thyroid-stimulating hormone (TSH) levels
  - Retinal examination through dilated pupils by an experienced examiner
  - Baseline electrocardiography (ECG) for adults aged >40 years, or aged >30 years with the presence of diabetes for >15 years, identified micro- or macrovascular complications, or other cardiac risk factors
  - Stress test/exercise ECG, if indicated by the presence of typical or atypical cardiac symptoms, associated vascular disease, or abnormalities on the baseline ECG (e.g., Q waves)

Monitoring diabetes

Evidenced-based diabetes targets have been determined for glycemic control and the prevention or delayed progression of long-term complications. Monitoring to assess those targets should be performed on a regular basis:

- A1C: every 3 months; the A1C value is determined by the 3-month lifespan of a red blood cell.
- Renal function, electrolytes, uACR, creatinine, eGFR: annually if normal and more often if abnormal or if management interventions are being undertaken.
- Lipid profile: annually if normal and more often if abnormal or if management interventions are being undertaken; liver function and/or creatinine kinase test if indicated by treatment interventions.
- Retinal assessment: every 2 years if normal and more often if abnormal or if management interventions are being undertaken.

DIABETES CARE: GLYCEMIC MANAGEMENT

Abstract

To achieve glycemic control of type 1 (T1) and type 2 (T2) diabetes, blood glucose and glycated hemoglobin targets have been established. Before the consideration of medications, effecting lifestyle changes in both nutritional and physical activity patterns provides the fundamentals of diabetes management. Details of nutritional approaches, from simple portion size tools to the more involved carbohydrate counting, are discussed. Insulin is used in T1 diabetes, whereas oral and/or parenteral antihyperglycemic medications and/or insulin will help achieve optimal glucose control in T2 diabetes. There are an increasing number of new noninsulin medications now available; their pharmacologic and clinical properties, including dosing, are reviewed. The variety of insulins currently available and their pharmacologic and clinical characteristics are also reviewed. Simple approaches to start and adjust insulin dosages are discussed.

Keywords: Antihyperglycemic agents (AHAs); Blood glucose targets; Glycated hemoglobin (A1C); Insulin starts and dosing; Lifestyle changes; Self-monitoring of blood glucose.

Practical Diabetes Care for Healthcare Professionals
ISBN 978-0-12-820082-7
https://doi.org/10.1016/B978-0-12-820082-7.00004-X

The fundamentals: lifestyle

Lifestyle changes remain the foundation upon which diabetes management is built. This is where diabetes management starts and is revisited often. By way of a disclaimer, I am not a Certified Diabetes Educator, dietitian, or nurse. What I describe throughout this book with respect to lifestyle changes by no means replaces the expert advice delivered by diabetes healthcare (DHC) team members. However, I hope to provide strategies that can be used in office situations to fill the gap until the DHC team becomes involved.

Skills
Self-monitoring of blood glucose

Self-monitoring of blood glucose (SMBG) provides useful educational feedback to people with diabetes. Understanding target blood glucose levels (Table 4.1) can help them assess the effect of their antihyperglycemic medication regimen and encourage them to change their nutritional intake and physical activity regimen to improve blood glucose control. Moreover, SMBG can motivate people to continue meeting the daily challenges that diabetes presents.

TABLE 4.1

Target A1C and blood glucose levels for adults

	A1C (%)	FPG/preprandial PG (mmol/L)	2-hour postprandial PG (mmol/L)
Target for most patients	$\leq$7.0	4.0–7.0	5.0–10.0
Normal range (consider for patients in whom it can be achieved safely)	$\leq$6.0	4.0–6.0	5.0–8.0

A1C, glycated hemoglobin; FPG, fasting plasma glucose; PG, plasma glucose.

For patients taking any antihyperglycemic agent (AHA) that has a higher risk for hypoglycemia, it is crucial that they continue SMBG to decrease that risk. As well, the use of any insulin regimen necessitates more frequent monitoring to evaluate its effect on glucose control and assess for risk of hypoglycemia.

SMBG frequency is truly at each patient's discretion. One practical regimen is to check once or twice per day, but at different times over the course of a given week (either before meals or 2 hours after meals). That way, over time, a person will be able to evaluate their diabetes control fairly well, recognize patterns of high or low blood glucose levels, and take steps to correct them.

Glycated hemoglobin

Glycated hemoglobin (A1C) is an effective and objective retrospective marker of blood glucose control over the previous 3 months. The A1C value is determined by the 3-month lifespan of a red blood cell. Although the recommended A1C target for most people with diabetes is ≤7.0%, this target can be individualized. Indeed, there will be circumstances where this target is too stringent, as attempting to achieve it may result in recurrent episodes of hypoglycemia. This must be considered in individuals who are vulnerable to hypoglycemia, in which case the target A1C can be relaxed to 7.5%–8.5%, depending on their circumstances (e.g., significant comorbidities, dependence on external caregivers).

Type 1 diabetes

While insulin is the mainstay management for type 1 (T1) diabetes, healthy lifestyle behaviors also improve T1 diabetes control. It is important for the person with T1 diabetes to be knowledgeable about balancing carbohydrate (CHO) intake, exercise, and insulin dosages. The person with T1 diabetes needs the complete DHC team to help learn about this balance, particularly the diabetes nurse educator and dietitian.

The DHC team will discuss the fundamental "survival skills" for T1 diabetes, including:

- Understanding T1 diabetes,
- How to perform SMBG,
- The different types of insulins (e.g., rapid and long acting) and how to administer them,
- How to recognize and treat hypoglycemia,
- Understanding CHO, including: What is CHO? What is the effect of CHO on blood glucose? What foods contain CHO and how much? How is the CHO content of foods calculated (aka CHO counting)?

Carbohydrate (CHO) counting

CHO counting is an important educational tool used in T1 and sometimes type 2 (T2) diabetes. People learn to measure the CHO content of foods and then calculate their mealtime rapid-acting insulin dose according to a predetermined insulin/CHO ratio to match or cover this CHO content. This method is best taught by diabetes educators, particularly the dietitian. There are numerous resources, both paper and online, to supplement the teaching. Some of these resources list the CHO content of mixed foods (e.g., casseroles), calculate the CHO content of recipes, list the CHO content in common restaurant foods, etc. Many popular restaurant chains list the CHO content of their menu items as well. It is even possible to purchase a nutritional scale that will determine the CHO content of foods at home.

There are different ways to approach CHO counting; however, the goal is to determine an individualized insulin/CHO ratio that can be used to calculate the rapid-acting insulin dose needed to cover a meal. Generally, 15 g CHO is the standard CHO "unit" or "choice" based on the concept that one uniform slice of bread contains 15 g of CHO. For example, if the insulin/CHO ratio is determined to be 1 unit/15 g CHO, then for a sandwich with two slices of bread the mealtime insulin dose will be calculated as 2 units.

Often, a correction factor (CF) is also determined as a way to add more insulin if the mealtime blood sugar is above target. For example, an individualized CF may be determined to be one extra unit of rapid-acting insulin for every 3.0 mmol/L blood sugar greater than the upper premeal target of 7.0 mmol/L. For the sandwich in the previous example, 2 units is the dose determined by the CHO content; however, if the premeal blood sugar is 10.0 mmol/L, then one extra unit is added as a CF making the total dose for the meal 3 units.

Additional adjustment is taught for exercise, where the preceding meal's insulin dose is decreased by 25%–50% for strenuous activity or exercise planned within 2 hours after the meal to prevent hypoglycemia.

Obviously, the person with T1 diabetes needs insulin from the time of diagnosis. The most common insulin regimen is termed "basal/bolus." "Basal" indicates a long-acting insulin given once or twice daily that will act continuously in the background, whereas "bolus" indicates a rapid-acting insulin that is given at mealtimes and possibly snacks to cover the glucose rise from CHO ingestion.

Further detailed information can be found in the section *Insulin: how to start*. The key is to refer a newly diagnosed person with T1 diabetes to an experienced DHC team in a timely fashion. Going forward, persons with T1 diabetes are best served in a shared care model, where the core DHC team includes an endocrinologist and the primary care provider along with the diabetes educators. Other healthcare professionals may be added as needed, e.g., optometrist, podiatrist or foot care nurse, pharmacist, etc.

Type 2 diabetes: where to start?

As the issue in T2 diabetes is a combination of insulin resistance and some degree of insulin deficiency, the benefit of adopting a healthy lifestyle can be very apparent for many people with T2 diabetes. Lifestyle changes, including eating healthy foods and exercising regularly, can result in significant improvements in glycemic control after a relatively short period. For those requiring medication, I like to think that following a healthy lifestyle will allow any AHA combination prescribed to have a better antiglycemic effect, i.e., "lifestyle changes give medications a fighting chance to work."

Lifestyle

Fundamental practical approaches can be made in the physician's office before the person with diabetes has the opportunity to participate in community-based diabetes education programs. Simple office strategies address the following.

• **Nutritional intake**

Perhaps the easiest and most efficient way to assess a person's nutritional intake is to review what they ate during the past 24 hours. This can be done quickly and it is often more revealing to ask "What did you *actually* eat?" rather than "What do you *usually* eat?"

It is very helpful to review quantities and sources of junk, snack, and fast foods, as well as sugar (regular soft drinks, unsweetened fruit juices, and even excessive quantities of milk all contain significant amounts of sugar). It is also useful to review portion sizes and dining habits away from home (e.g., how often do you eat fast food or visit restaurants and buffets?).

There are some easy tools to teach appropriate portion size, including the plate method and the handy portion guide (Figs. 4.1 and 4.2).

• **Diets**

For those individuals who are seeking a diet, there is evidence that some dietary patterns help lower blood glucose levels and contribute to weight loss. Some examples include the Mediterranean diet, a vegetarian or vegan diet and the DASH (Dietary Approaches to Stop Hypertension) diet. All these nutritional approaches emphasize eating patterns that are rich in vegetables, fruit, whole grains, and lower-fat proteins (e.g., poultry, fish, and pulses such as beans, lentils, and chickpeas).

Fad diets

A new "fad" diet seems to become popular every few months. These diets range from the original "liquid protein" diets through Atkins, South Beach, Zone, Blood Type, and Paleo to the most current Ketogenic and Intermittent Fasting diets. Most seem to adhere to the principle of low or even no CHO intake. Although they

Plate method to determine portion size

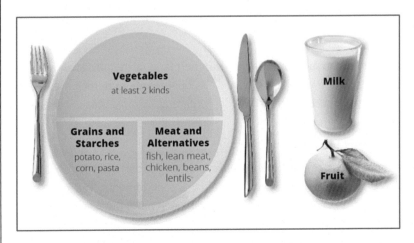

Vegetables
at least 2 kinds

Milk

Grains and
Starches
potato, rice,
corn, pasta

Meat and
Alternatives
fish, lean meat,
chicken, beans,
lentils·

Fruit

Source: Reproduced with permission from Diabetes Canada 2018 Clinical Practice Guidelines for the Prevention and Management of Diabetes in Canada.

are often successful in the short term, they are very difficult to sustain over the long term. The problem arises when a person follows one of these diets and loses weight but cannot sustain the diet and regains the lost weight and often more. This results in a "yo-yo" diet cycle, which is extremely unhealthy.

- **Physical activity**

Often, emphasis is placed on the "diet" part of diabetes management, overlooking the fact that regular physical activity is also a key factor in the healthy lifestyle approach to diabetes management. During the initial assessment, establish if the person is active outside their normal daily activities (being busy at work does not count!).

Walking is the simplest and least expensive way to start a physical activity regimen. Does the person have adequate running or walking shoes and somewhere safe to walk, especially in winter?

When advising physical activity, start small; walking for 10–15 minutes twice daily seems more manageable if a person has not walked in years. Can they ultimately aim for 30–60 minutes each day? What are the barriers to physical activity and how can they be overcome? Often, the person's state of mind or readiness to change presents the greatest challenge.

FIGURE 4.2

Handy portion guide to determine portion size

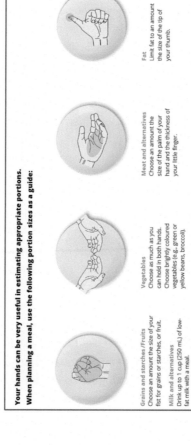

**Your hands can be very useful in estimating appropriate portions.
When planning a meal, use the following portion sizes as a guide:**

Grains and starches/Fruits
Choose an amount the size of your
fist for grains or starches, or fruit.

Milk and alternatives
Drink up to 1 cup (250 mL) of low-
fat milk with a meal.

Vegetables
Choose as much as you
can hold in both hands.
Choose brightly coloured
vegetables (e.g., green or
yellow beans, broccoli).

Meat and alternatives
Choose an amount the
size of the palm of your
hand and the thickness of
your little finger.

Fat
Limit fat to an amount
the size of the tip of
your thumb.

Source: Reproduced with permission from Diabetes Canada 2018 Clinical Practice Guidelines for the Prevention and Management of Diabetes in Canada.

Management of type 2 diabetes: antihyperglycemic agents
When to add medications

To reiterate, all people with diabetes benefit from diabetes education, especially with respect to nutritional intake and physical activity. Although behavior changes take time, even small changes can improve clinical outcomes. However, in the presence of significant hyperglycemia, it is important to start medications at the same time that lifestyle changes are being addressed.

What is significant hyperglycemia? By consensus, an A1C of 8.5% represents the cutoff. The decision regarding whether and when to initiate or add medications should be based on glycemic control. If glycemic control is poor (generally deemed to be A1C >8.5%), then medication (either single or combination therapy) should be started while lifestyle changes are initiated. If the person is clinically thought to be metabolically decompensating with significant symptoms of hyperglycemia, unexplained weight loss, or signs of an acute complication such as diabetic ketoacidosis (DKA) or hyperglycemic hyperosmolar nonketotic state (HHNK), then insulin should be initiated from the beginning with or without AHAs.

Timely reassessment will help determine the need to start or add medications in order to achieve target A1C and blood glucose levels (Table 4.1).

The choice of AHA should be determined on an individual basis. A basic knowledge of the mechanisms of action of the various AHA categories is necessary. The general approach is to evaluate AHAs, singly or in combination, based on their ability to decrease and maintain A1C levels in the context of their safety, tolerability, ease of use, and cost.

Most often, an insulin sensitizer (i.e., metformin) is the first-line agent. Combinations of AHAs in submaximal dosages can result in more rapid and improved glycemic control. AHAs may be used effectively in combination with insulin—often basal insulin—or, depending on the mechanism of action of the AHA, along with premeal rapid-acting bolus insulin and basal insulin.

Current evidence shows that lower blood glucose levels at the time of initiation of therapy are associated with lower A1C levels over time and decreased long-term complications. Accordingly, a patient will have better long-term diabetes control if the treatment intervention is initiated early when the metabolic abnormalities of diabetes are usually less severe.

Management of type 2 diabetes: general approaches

- For A1C <8.5%, lifestyle ± 1 AHA can be initiated. Metformin remains the recommended first choice of agent.
- For A1C ≥8.5%, combination therapy using two AHAs should be considered. Recommended options are metformin plus another of the following listed AHAs.
  - However, current evidence recommends that in the presence of cardiovascular disease (CVD), consideration should be given to either a sodium glucose co-transporter 2 (SGLT2) inhibitor or a glucagon-like peptide 1 (GLP-1) receptor agonist of the incretin class as the second choice.

Antihyperglycemic agents available in type 2 diabetes management

1. Metformin
   - Renal function must be assessed before recommending metformin. In the presence of reduced renal function (defined as serum creatinine >130 µmol/L or estimated glomerular filtration rate [eGFR] <60 mL/min/1.73 m^2), metformin should be kept to a maximum dose of 500 mg bid. In the presence of worsening renal function with a serum creatinine >160 µmol/L or eGFR <30 mL/min/1.73 m^2, metformin should not be administered.
2. Insulin secretagogues
   - Generally, gliclazide is chosen over glyburide because it carries less risk for hypoglycemia and is available in a convenient once-daily formulation.
3. Incretin agents
   - Dipeptidyl peptidase-4 (DPP-4) inhibitors (sitagliptin, saxagliptin, or linagliptin).
   - GLP-1 receptor agonists (liraglutide or exenatide as daily formulations or dulaglutide, semaglutide or exenatide extended release as weekly formulations).

While the oral members of the incretin class, DPP-4 inhibitors, appear to be useful, the GLP-1 receptor agonists, which are parenteral, have now been shown to provide CVD and renal benefits [1–4]. The incretin class, particularly GLP-1 receptor agonists, may aid in weight loss. However, concerns about the relationship between incretins and pancreatic inflammation or possible malignant changes (pancreatic and medullary carcinoma of the thyroid) make a thorough clinical assessment important before initiating therapy. It is important to remember that, to date, no significant warnings have been reported for this medication class.

4. SGLT2 inhibitors (canagliflozin, empagliflozin, dapagliflozin, ertugliflozin).
   • This newer class of AHA is increasingly being shown to be effective in lowering blood glucose levels and possibly aiding in weight loss. Importantly, this class has now been shown to have both CVD benefits, particularly in those individuals with identified CVD, and renal protective benefits [5–10]. Concerns include frequency of genital urinary mycotic infections, rarely perineal infections (necrotizing fasciitis or Fournier's gangrene), and, more importantly, a slightly increased risk of euglycemic DKA.
5. Meglitinide, a short-acting insulin secretagogue (target is postprandial hyperglycemia only).
6. α1-Glucosidase inhibitor, which blunts gastrointestinal polysaccharide absorption (target is postprandial hyperglycemia only).
7. Thiazolidinediones (TZDs), which decrease insulin resistance, may play a limited role in diabetes.
   • Evidence linking the TZDs, rosiglitazone in particular, to cardiac events has decreased their usage. There still may be a role for pioglitazone in the management of prediabetes or early mild diabetes in people with no history or risk factor profile for CVD. Rosiglitazone cannot be prescribed without both a physician and patient waiver.

Remember, it is important to reassess patients in a timely manner, within 4–6 weeks. If glycemic control is not within or approaching target, then reassess lifestyle factors as well, and consider adding another agent(s) and/or basal insulin. Aggressive combination therapy from the onset of newly diagnosed diabetes, particularly with A1C >8.5%, including the use of basal insulin, has been shown to be effective.

Table 4.2 summarizes the AHAs currently available in Canada, their general mechanisms of action, dosage and dosing strategies, and common adverse effects.

Fig. 4.3 outlines the dosage adjustment required in the presence of decreased renal function. It is a very useful figure for quick reference.

Management of type 1 or type 2 diabetes: insulin
Table 4.3 lists the currently available types of insulin by their time action profiles.

Fig. 4.4 depicts rapid- and long-acting insulin action profiles.

Insulin: how to start
Refer to Table 4.1 for target blood glucose levels.

TABLE 4.2

Antihyperglycemic agents

Agent	Mechanism of action	Dosage	Action time	Benefits	Disadvantages
Biguanide (insulin sensitizer)					
Metformin (Glucophage)	• Insulin sensitizer • Reduces hepatic glucose output	• Start 250–500 mg bid ac meals • Start with low dose and increase slowly • Maximum dose 2550 mg/day in divided doses	8 hours	• Does not promote weight gain • Rarely causes hypoglycemia • Can be used in combination with daytime insulin	• GI: nausea, bloating, diarrhea • Slow increase in dose decreases these side effects: "start low, go slow" • Contraindicated in renal impairment (eGFR <30 mL/min/1.73 m^2), hepatic impairment, or CHF • Maximum dose of 500 mg bid with eGFR 30–60 mL/min/1.73 m^2
Sulfonylureas (insulin secretagogues)					
Glyburide (Diabeta, Glibenclamide)	• Stimulates pancreatic secretion of insulin	• Start at 2.5–5 mg od or bid ac meals • Maximum dose, 10 mg bid	16–24 hours	• Sulfonylureas are often the most potent AHA class	• May cause weight gain • May cause hypoglycemia

Continued

TABLE 4.2

Antihyperglycemic agents—cont'd

Agent	Mechanism of action	Dosage	Action time	Benefits	Disadvantages
Gliclazide (Diamicron)	• Stimulates pancreatic secretion of insulin	• Start at 80 mg od • Maximum dose, 160 mg bid	8–16 hours	• Causes less hypoglycemia than glyburide	• May cause weight gain
Gliclazide MR (Diamicron MR)	• Stimulates pancreatic secretion of insulin	• Start at 30 mg od • Maximum dose, 120 mg od	24 hours	• Causes less hypoglycemia than glyburide	• May cause weight gain
Glimepiride (Amaryl)	• Stimulates pancreatic secretion of insulin	• Start at 1–2 mg od • Dosage range: 1–8 mg od	24 hours	• May be used in combination with daytime insulin • May cause less hypoglycemia than glyburide	• May cause weight gain
α-Glucosidase inhibitor					
Acarbose (Prandase, Glucobay)	• Inhibits glucosidase enzymes in CHO digestion • Decreases postprandial glucose rise	• Start at 25 mg with first bite of food • Titrate weekly to usual dose of 50–100 mg/meal	Best effect seen postprandially	• No hypoglycemia if used alone	• GI: bloating, flatus • Start with low dose and increase slowly to decrease GI side effects • Beano counteracts glucose effects • When treating hypoglycemia use dextrose tablets, milk, or honey

Meglitinide (insulin secretagogue)

Repaglinide (GlucoNorm)	• Stimulates pancreatic insulin secretion • Different mechanisms of action than sulfonylureas	• Start at 0.5 mg 0–30 minutes before each meal • Or titrate according to CHO intake (1 mg/15 g CHO) • Available in 0.5, 1, and 2 mg dosages	Short-acting; stimulates insulin secretion in response to glucose rise at mealtime	• Controls postprandial glucose rise • Provides flexibility to fit varied mealtimes	• May cause hypoglycemia

Thiazolidinediones (insulin sensitizers)

Rosiglitazone (Avandia)	• Insulin sensitizer • Insulin action improved in liver, muscle, and adipose tissue	• 2–8 mg daily as a bid dosage	Effect seen after 6 weeks	• May increase TG and decrease HDL levels	• May cause weight gain, peripheral edema, macular edema, or CHF • Rare occurrence of osteoporosis in women • Contraindicated in CHF, hepatic impairment (monitor liver function test results regularly) • Should not be used in combination with daytime insulin • Rosiglitazone, alone or in combination, is prescribed with both physician and patient waivers

Continued

TABLE 4.2

Antihyperglycemic agents—cont'd

Agent	Mechanism of action	Dosage	Action time	Benefits	Disadvantages
Rosiglitazone/metformin (Avandamet)	• As per rosiglitazone and metformin	• Rosiglitazone: 1—4 mg • Metformin: 500—1000 mg	4—6 weeks	• As per rosiglitazone and metformin	• As per rosiglitazone and metformin
Rosiglitazone/glimepiride (Avandaryl)	• As per rosiglitazone and glimepiride	• Rosiglitazone: 1—4 mg • Glimepiride: 1, 2, or 4 mg	4—6 weeks	• As per rosiglitazone and glimepiride	• As per rosiglitazone and glimepiride
Pioglitazone (Actos)	• Insulin sensitizer • Insulin action improved in liver, muscle, and adipose tissue	• 15—45 mg daily	4—6 weeks	• As per rosiglitazone	• As per rosiglitazone • May be associated with a risk of bladder cancer • Does not require waiver for prescription

Pioglitazone/ metformin (Actoplus Met)	• As per pioglitazone and metformin	• Pioglitazone: 15 mg • Metformin: 500 and 850 mg	4–6 weeks	• As per pioglitazone and metformin	• As per pioglitazone and metformin
Pioglitazone/ glimepiride (Duetact)	• As per metformin and glimepiride	• Pioglitazone: 30 mg • Glimepiride: 2 and 4 mg	4–6 weeks	• As per pioglitazone and glimepiride	• As per pioglitazone and glimepiride
Incretins (augment insulin action)					
Sitagliptin (Januvia)	• Augments endogenous insulin • Blocks glucagon action in liver • Sensitizer and secretagogue effects	• 100 mg daily (50 mg daily with renal impairment)	4–6 weeks	• Weight neutral • Low risk for hypoglycemia	• Rare risk of pancreatitis • Contraindicated in those with a history of medullary thyroid cancer/ multiple endocrine neoplasia • Requires dosage reduction in the presence of CKD

Continued

TABLE 4.2

Antihyperglycemic agents—cont'd

Agent	Mechanism of action	Dosage	Action time	Benefits	Disadvantages
Sitagliptin/ metformin (Janumet)	• As per sitagliptin and metformin	• Sitagliptin: 50 mg • Metformin: 500—1000 mg	As per sitagliptin and metformin	• As per sitagliptin and metformin	• As per sitagliptin and metformin
Saxagliptin (Onglyza)	• Augments endogenous insulin • Blocks glucagon action in liver • Sensitizer and secretagogue effects	• 5 mg daily	4—6 weeks	• Weight neutral	• Rare risk of pancreatitis • Contraindicated in those with a history of medullary thyroid cancer/ multiple endocrine neoplasia • Requires dosage reduction in the presence of CKD
Saxagliptin/ metformin (Kombiglyze)	• As per saxagliptin and metformin	• Saxagliptin: 2.5, 5 mg • Metformin: 500 and 1000 mg	4—6 weeks	• As per saxagliptin and metformin	• As per saxagliptin and metformin

| Linagliptin (Trajenta) | • Augments endogenous insulin
• Blocks glucagon action in liver
• Sensitizer and secretagogue effects | • 5 mg daily | 4–6 weeks | • Does not require dosage adjustment in the presence of CKD | • Rare risk of pancreatitis
• Contraindicated in those with a history of medullary thyroid cancer/multiple endocrine neoplasia
• No dosage reduction until an eGFR of 15 mL/min/1.73 m^2 |
| Linagliptin/ metformin (Jentadueto) | • Augments endogenous insulin
• Blocks glucagon action in liver
• Sensitizer and secretagogue effects | • Linagliptin: 2.5 mg
• Metformin: 500, 850, and 1000 mg | 4–6 weeks | • Does not require dosage adjustment in the presence of CKD | • As per linagliptin and metformin |

Continued

TABLE 4.2

Antihyperglycemic agents—cont'd

Agent	Mechanism of action	Dosage	Action time	Benefits	Disadvantages
GLP-1 receptor agonists (augment endogenous insulin)					
Liraglutide (Victoza)	• Augments endogenous insulin • Blocks glucagon action in liver • Sensitizer and secretagogue effects	0.6—1.8 sc mg daily	4—6 weeks	• Weight neutral • May lead to weight loss • Indications for CVD and renal benefits	• May cause nausea • Rare risk of pancreatitis • Contraindicated in those with a history of medullary thyroid cancer/ multiple endocrine neoplasia • Not advised when eGFR <15 mL/min/ 1.73 m^2
Lixisenatide daily (Adlyxine)	• Augments endogenous insulin • Blocks glucagon action in liver • Sensitizer and secretagogue effects	10 μg sc od for 14 days then titrate to maintenance dose of 20 μg od	4—6 weeks	• Weight neutral • May lead to weight loss	• May cause nausea • Rare risk of pancreatitis • Contraindicated in those with a history of medullary thyroid cancer/ multiple endocrine neoplasia • Contraindicated when eGFR <30 mL/min/ 1.73 m^2

Exenatide (extended release) (Bydureon)	• Augments endogenous insulin • Blocks glucagon action in liver • Sensitizer and secretagogue effects	2 mg sc weekly	4–6 weeks	• Weight neutral • May lead to weight loss	• May cause nausea • Rare risk of pancreatitis • Contraindicated in those with a history of medullary thyroid cancer/multiple endocrine neoplasia • Caution when eGFR <50 mL/min/1.73 m^2 and stop if eGFR <30 mL/min/1.73 m^2
Dulaglutide weekly (Trulicity)	• Augments endogenous insulin • Blocks glucagon action in liver • Sensitizer and secretagogue effects	0.75 mg weekly, which can be titrated to 1.5 mg weekly after 1–2 weeks	4–6 weeks	• Weight neutral • May lead to weight loss • Indications for CVD and renal benefits	• May cause nausea • Rare risk of pancreatitis • Contraindicated in those with a history of medullary thyroid cancer/multiple endocrine neoplasia • Caution when eGFR <15 mL/min/1.73 m^2

Continued

TABLE 4.2

Antihyperglycemic agents—cont'd

Agent	Mechanism of action	Dosage	Action time	Benefits	Disadvantages
Semaglutide weekly (Ozempic)	• Augments endogenous insulin • Blocks glucagon action in liver • Sensitizer and secretagogue effects	• 0.25 mg sc weekly • After 4 weeks the dose should be increased to 0.5 mg sc weekly • Additional titration may be increased to 1 mg once weekly	4–6 weeks	• Weight neutral • May lead to weight loss • Shown to have CVD and renal benefits	• May cause nausea • Rare risk of pancreatitis • Contraindicated in those with a history of medullary thyroid cancer/multiple endocrine neoplasia • Caution when eGFR <15 mL/min/1.73 m^2
Semaglutide daily (Rybelsus)	• Augments endogenous insulin • Blocks glucagon action in liver • Sensitizer and secretagogue effects	• 3 mg po daily • After 30 days may increase to 7 mg po daily • Additional titration to 14 mg daily may be increased after another 30 days	4–6 weeks	• Oral medication • Weight neutral • May lead to weight loss • May also have CVD and renal benefits	• May cause nausea • Rare risk of pancreatitis • Contraindicated in those with past history of medullary thyroid cancer/multiple endocrine neoplasia • Caution when eGFR <15 mL/min/1.73 m^2

SGLT2 inhibitors

Canagliflozin (Invokana)	• Inhibits renal reabsorption of glucose	• 100–300 mg daily	4–6 weeks	• May cause modest weight loss • Indications for CVD and renal benefits • Now indicated to continue in patients with eGFR ≥15 mL/min/1.73 m²	• Glycosuria may increase risk of GU mycotic infections • Rare risk of perineal infections • Risk of dehydration, particularly in elderly and/or in those who use diuretics • Rare risk of euglycemic DKA, should be discontinued with intercurrent illness • Earlier study indicating increased risk of toe amputation but not confirmed in later study • Not advised when eGFR <15 mL/min/1.73 m²
Canagliflozin/ Metformin (Invokamet)	• As per canagliflozin and metformin	• Canagliflozin: 50 and 150 mg • Metformin: 500 and 1000 mg	4–6 weeks	• As per canagliflozin and metformin	• As per canagliflozin and metformin
Dapagliflozin (Forxiga)	• Inhibits renal reabsorption of glucose	• 5–10 mg daily	6 weeks	• May cause modest weight loss • Shown to have benefits in congestive heart failure	• Glycosuria may increase risk of GU mycotic infections • Rare risk of perineal infections • Risk of dehydration, particularly in elderly and/or in those who use diuretics

Continued

TABLE 4.2

Antihyperglycemic agents—cont'd

Agent	Mechanism of action	Dosage	Action time	Benefits	Disadvantages
					• Rare risk of euglycemic DKA, should be discontinued with intercurrent illness • Caution with decreased renal function
Dapagliflozin/ metformin (Xigduo)	• As per dapagliflozin and metformin	• Dapagliflozin: 5 and 10 mg • Metformin: 500 and 1000 mg	4—6 weeks	• As per dapagliflozin and metformin	• As per dapagliflozin and metformin
Empagliflozin (Jardiance)	• Inhibits renal reabsorption of glucose	• 10—25 mg daily	4—6 weeks	• May cause modest weight loss • Indications for CVD and renal benefit	• Glycosuria may increase risk of GU mycotic infections • Rare risk of perineal infections • Risk of dehydration, particularly in elderly and/or in those who use diuretics • Rare risk of euglycemic DKA, should be discontinued with intercurrent illness • Caution with decreased renal function

Drug	Mechanism	Dose	Time	Benefits	Adverse effects/warnings
Empagliflozin/ metformin (Synjardy)	• As per empagliflozin and metformin	• Empagliflozin: 5 and 12.5 mg • Metformin: 500 and 1000 mg	4–6 weeks	• As per empagliflozin and metformin	• As per empagliflozin and metformin
Empagliflozin/ metformin extended release (Synjardy XR)	• As per empagliflozin and metformin	• Empagliflozin: 5, 10, and 12.5 mg • Metformin: 1000 mg	4–6 weeks	• As per empagliflozin and metformin	• As per empagliflozin and metformin
Ertugliflozin (Steglatro)	• Inhibits renal reabsorption of glucose	• 5–15 mg daily	4–6 weeks	• May cause modest weight loss • No evidence yet for CVD or renal benefits	• Glycosuria may increase risk of GU mycotic infections • Rare risk of perineal infections • Risk of dehydration, particularly in elderly and/or in those who use diuretics • Rare risk of euglycemic DKA, should be discontinued with intercurrent illness • Contraindicated when eGFR <45 mL/min/ 1.73 m^2

Continued

TABLE 4.2

Antihyperglycemic agents—cont'd

Agent	Mechanism of action	Dosage	Action time	Benefits	Disadvantages
Sotagliflozin (Zynquista in the European Union; not yet approved in North America)	• As per ertugliflozin	• 200–400 mg OD	• 4–6 weeks	• Recent studies have indicated possible benefit for CVD and hospitalization for congestive heart failure	• Glycosuria may increase risk of GU mycotic infections • Rare risk of perineal infections • Risk of dehydration, particularly in elderly and/or in those who use diuretics • Rare risk of euglycemic DKA, should be discontinued with intercurrent illness • Caution with decreased renal function
Dopamine agonist (novel use for diabetes)					
Bromocriptine-QR (Cycloset)		• 0.8 mg daily, titrated weekly to 1.6–4.8 mg			• Nausea • Postural dizziness
Weight loss agent					
Orlistat (Xenical)	• Inhibits lipase	• 100 mg with each meal			• Adverse GI effects

Insulin/AHA combinations

			1–2 weeks	• As per lixisenatide and glargine	• As per lixisenatide and glargine
Insulin glargine/ lixisenatide (Soliqua)	Lixisenatide actions: • Augments endogenous insulin • Blocks glucagon action in liver • Therefore both sensitizer and secretagogue effects Glargine actions: • Refer to insulin section	• Therapy with basal insulin should be discontinued prior to initiation of Soliqua • In patients inadequately controlled on <30 units of basal insulin, the recommended starting dosage of Soliqua is 15 units (15 units glargine/ 5 µg lixisenatide) given sc once daily • Titration according to FPG by 2–4 units insulin/week • Titration of insulin automatically changes lixisenatide dose			

Continued

TABLE 4.2

Antihyperglycemic agents—cont'd

Agent	Mechanism of action	Dosage	Action time	Benefits	Disadvantages
Insulin degludec/ liraglutide (Xultophy)	Liraglutide actions: • Augments endogenous insulin • Blocks glucagon action in liver • Therefore both sensitizer and secretagogue effects Degludec actions: • Refer to insulin section	• Basal insulin therapy should be discontinued prior to initiation of Xultophy • In patients inadequately controlled on <50 units of basal insulin or liraglutide (≤1.8 g daily) the recommended starting dosage is as follows: • New start: 10 units of insulin degludec and 0.36 mg liraglutide • Converting from basal insulin or liraglutide: 16 units of insulin degludec and 0.58 mg liraglutide	1–2 weeks	• As per liraglutide and degludec	• As per liraglutide and degludec

	• Dose may be titrated twice/weekly by 1–2 units of insulin as the liraglutide will automatically change according to FPG to a maximum of 50/1.8 mg

ac, before meals; *AHA*, antihyperglycemic agent; *bid*, twice daily; *CHF*, congestive heart failure; *CHO*, carbohydrate; *CKD*, chronic kidney disease; *CVD*, cardiovascular disease; *DKA*, diabetic ketoacidosis; *eGFR*, estimated glomerular filtration rate; *FPG*, fasting plasma glucose; *GI*, gastrointestinal; *GLP-1*, glucagon-like peptide 1; *GU*, genitourinary; *HDL*, high-density lipoprotein; *od*, once daily; *sc*, subcutaneously; *SGLT2*, sodium glucose co-transporter 2; *TG*, triglyceride; *tid*, three times daily.

FIGURE 4.3

Antihyperglycemic agents and dose adjustment for renal function

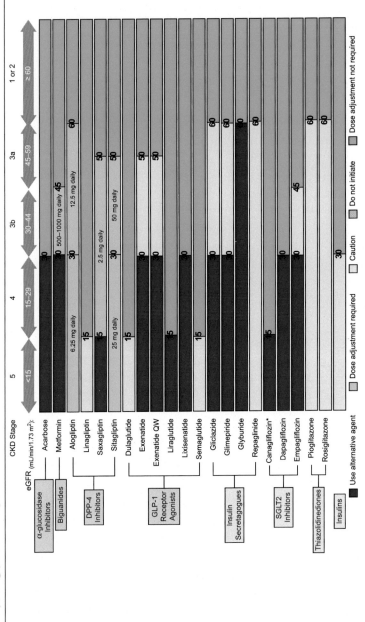

Source: Reproduced with permission from Diabetes Canada 2018 Clinical Practice Guidelines for the Prevention and Management of Diabetes in Canada.
CKD, chronic kidney disease; CVD, cardiovascular disease; DPP-4, dipeptidyl peptidase-4; eGFR, estimated glomerular filtration rate; GLP-1, glucagon-like peptide 1;
SGLT2, sodium glucose co-transporter 2.

TABLE 4.3

Insulin types

Type	Trade name	Onset	Peak	Duration
Rapid-acting (analogue)				
Aspart, ultrarapid-acting Lispro (U-100 or U-200) Aspart Glulisine	Fiasp Humalog NovoRapid Apidra	4–5 minutes 10–15 minutes 10–15 minutes 10–15 minutes	1.0–1.5 hours	2–4 hours
Short-acting (human)				
Regular	Humulin R Novolin ge Toronto	0.5–1 hours	2–4 hours	6–8 hours
Intermediate-acting (human)				
NPH	Humulin N	1–3 hours	4–8 hours	12–16 hours
Long-acting (analogue)				
Glargine U-300 glargine Detemir Degludec (U-100 or U-200)	Lantus Toujeo Levemir Tresiba	90 minutes	No peak	24 hours >24 hours

Continued

TABLE 4.3

Insulin types—cont'd

Type	Trade name	Onset	Peak	Duration
Premixed (short- and intermediate-acting, R/NPH) (human)				
30/70 40/60 50/50	Humulin (30/70 only) Novolin ge	0.5 hours	2—12 hours 2—3 hours 1 hour	12—18 hours
Premixed insulin (rapid- and intermediate-acting) (analogue)				
25% rapid-acting/75% intermediate-acting 30% rapid-acting/70% intermediate-acting 50% rapid-acting/50% intermediate-acting	Humalog Mix 25 NovoMix 70/30 Mix 50	15 minutes	90 minutes—4 hours	10—14 hours

NPH, neutral protamine Hagedorn; R, regular insulin.

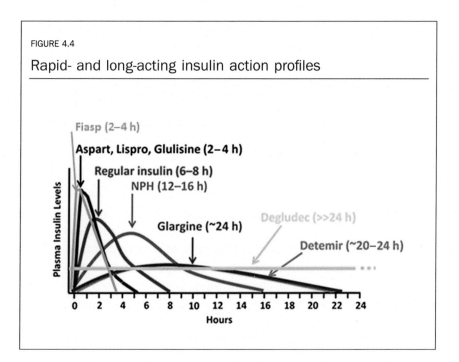

FIGURE 4.4

Rapid- and long-acting insulin action profiles

- **Basal insulin**
    - For the person who is not insulin resistant (i.e., not overweight) start with 5 units at bedtime (hs).
    - For the person considered insulin resistant (i.e., overweight) start with 10 units at bedtime (hs).
    - Titrate insulin dose by 1–2 units every 3 days until blood glucose targets are met in the morning.
    - Alternatively, insulin can be started on a weight basis, starting at 0.2–0.3 units/kg for the total daily dose (TDD).
    - Generally, 50% of the TDD of insulin consists of basal insulin.
    - Some people prefer to take their basal insulin at suppertime or in the morning, instead of at bedtime.
    - Generally, the newer long-acting insulin analogues are preferable to NPH.

- **Bolus insulin**
    - If the person is CHO counting start with 1 unit/15 g CHO at mealtimes.
    - People may require different insulin/CHO ratios for different meals, e.g., breakfast, 2 units/15 g CHO; lunch, 1 unit/15 g CHO; and supper, 3 units/15 g CHO.

- If the person is not CHO counting, then a "flat" dose of rapid-acting insulin can be determined after a dietitian-initiated assessment of the average CHO intake at each meal.
- The starting dose of rapid-acting insulin can be titrated every 1–2 days until blood glucose targets (either 2 hours after the meal or before the next meal) are met.
- A CF is the extra insulin given at mealtime to "correct" for premeal blood sugars over target. The CF is individually determined, often starting with one extra unit of rapid-acting insulin for every 3.0 mmol/L blood sugar >7.0 mmol/L. This CF is added to the assessed mealtime rapid-acting insulin dose. It is not recommended to administer a CF dose at bedtime, as it may increase the risk of nocturnal hypoglycemia. If the CF is consistently required, then the mealtime bolus dose of insulin should be adjusted.
- Effectiveness of the insulin/CHO ratio can be assessed by checking blood glucose values 2 hours after meals to determine whether glucose targets have been met (Table 4.1).
- Generally, 50% of the TDD of insulin is bolus, divided among the usual three meals.
- Snacks:
  - If <30 g CHO, often no insulin is needed
  - If ≥30 g CHO, then usually one-half of the mealtime insulin/CHO ratio is recommended
- Bolus insulin dosage is generally decreased by 25–50% when vigorous exercise/activity is anticipated within 2 hours of the meal to prevent hypoglycemia.

Insulin/antihyperglycemic agent combinations

These combinations can be used for the management of T2 diabetes.

• Bedtime insulin and antihyperglycemic agents

Introducing insulin at bedtime is a relatively simple method to add insulin to a combination regimen with AHAs. Basal insulin is added at bedtime to help counteract hepatic glucose output during the night and thus lower fasting plasma glucose (FPG) in the morning. Starting the day with a lower FPG level will allow the AHAs taken during the day to be more effective.

The insulin regimens outlined in the following are listed in the order in which they are commonly administered in T2 diabetes. However, any regimen may be chosen, depending on individual circumstances. Figs. 4.5—4.9 illustrate the various insulin/AHA combinations that can be used.

FIGURE 4.5

Bedtime insulin and antihyperglycemic agents

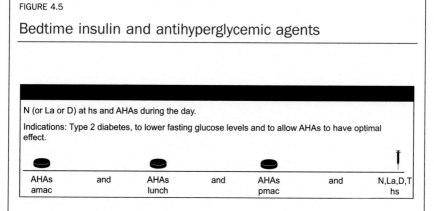

N (or La or D) at hs and AHAs during the day.

Indications: Type 2 diabetes, to lower fasting glucose levels and to allow AHAs to have optimal effect.

| AHAs amac | and | AHAs lunch | and | AHAs pmac | and | N,La,D,T hs |

amac, before breakfast; *D*, detemir insulin; *hs*, bedtime; *La*, glargine insulin; *N*, NPH insulin; *T*, degludec insulin; *pmac*, before supper.

- **Notes**
  - Start with ≤5 units hs if the person is lean, or ≥10 units hs if the person is not lean.
  - Alternatively, calculate the starting insulin dosage by 0.2—0.3 units/kg.
  - Titrate the dosage according to FPG by 1—2 units every 3 days until the target FPG is met.
  - Rapid-acting insulin CF: start with 1 unit for every 3.0 mmol/L >7.0 mmol/L; can be used at meals along with AHAs.

- **Daytime insulin and antihyperglycemic agents**

Once- or twice-daily basal insulin can be used with most AHAs during the day in effective combinations (Fig. 4.6).

FIGURE 4.6

Daytime insulin (generally NPH) and antihyperglycemic agents

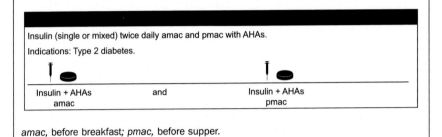

Insulin (single or mixed) twice daily amac and pmac with AHAs.

Indications: Type 2 diabetes.

| Insulin + AHAs
amac | and | Insulin + AHAs
pmac |

amac, before breakfast; *pmac,* before supper.

- **Notes**
  - Long-acting analogue or intermediate-acting insulin; the second dose may be given at bedtime, rather than at supper.
  - Initial dosage: ≤5 units bid if person is lean or ≥10 units bid if person is not lean.
  - Alternatively, calculate the starting dosage by 0.2–0.3 units/kg.
  - Titrate the dosage according to SMBG, FPG, and presupper blood glucose levels by 1–2 units every 3 days until blood glucose is at target.

- **Basal/bolus insulin**

The term "basal/bolus insulin" is a more functional term than the commonly used "multiple dose insulin," as it describes more precisely the insulin regimen. Although this is the sole regimen used for T1 diabetes, it can also be used in T2 diabetes (Fig. 4.7).

FIGURE 4.7

Basal/bolus insulin: four times daily

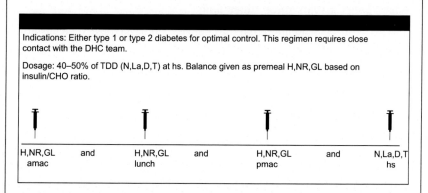

Indications: Either type 1 or type 2 diabetes for optimal control. This regimen requires close contact with the DHC team.

Dosage: 40–50% of TDD (N,La,D,T) at hs. Balance given as premeal H,NR,GL based on insulin/CHO ratio.

| H,NR,GL | and | H,NR,GL | and | H,NR,GL | and | N,La,D,T |
| amac | | lunch | | pmac | | hs |

amac, before breakfast; *CHO*, carbohydrate; *D*, detemir insulin; *DHC*, diabetes healthcare; *GL*, glulisine; *H*, lispro insulin; *hs*, bedtime; *La*, glargine insulin; *N*, NPH insulin; *T*, degludec insulin; *NR*, insulin aspart; *pmac*, before supper; *TDD*, total daily dose.

- **Notes**
  - TDD should be calculated as indicated later for basal and bolus insulin.
  - Alternatively, TDD can be calculated as 0.2–0.3 units/kg to start.

Basal insulin
  - If starting as a new regimen, initial dosage is ≤5 units bid if person is lean or ≥10 units bid if person is not lean.
  - Alternatively, calculate the starting dosage by using 50% of the calculated TDD.
  - Titrate the dosage of basal insulin according to the FPG by 1–2 units every 3 days until the target FPG is met.

Rapid-acting insulin
  - Rapid-acting insulin dosage may be determined by the insulin/CHO ratio, starting with 1 unit rapid-acting insulin/15 g CHO.
  - Alternatively, the rapid-acting insulin dosage may be determined as a "flat dosage" for each meal based on an average CHO intake for each meal, calculating 1 unit/15 g CHO to begin.

- CF for rapid-acting insulin: 1—2 units for every 3.0 mmol/L >7.0 mmol/L at meals only; a CF dose is *not* recommended at night if the person is using a long-acting analogue, as this increases the risk for nocturnal hypoglycemia.

- **Basal/bolus insulin: three times daily**

This is an alternative regimen that may help patients who have difficulty fitting in the lunchtime bolus insulin dose (Fig. 4.8).

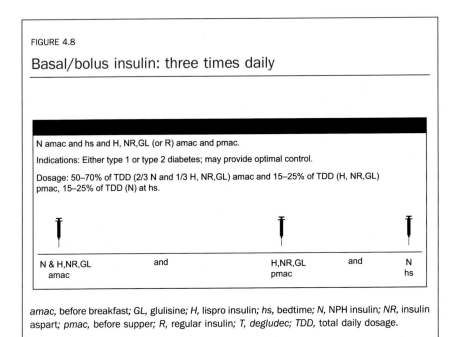

FIGURE 4.8

Basal/bolus insulin: three times daily

N amac and hs and H, NR,GL (or R) amac and pmac.

Indications: Either type 1 or type 2 diabetes; may provide optimal control.

Dosage: 50–70% of TDD (2/3 N and 1/3 H, NR,GL) amac and 15–25% of TDD (H, NR,GL) pmac, 15–25% of TDD (N) at hs.

| N & H,NR,GL amac | and | H,NR,GL pmac | and | N hs |

amac, before breakfast; *GL*, glulisine; *H*, lispro insulin; *hs*, bedtime; *N*, NPH insulin; *NR*, insulin aspart; *pmac*, before supper; *R*, regular insulin; *T*, degludec; *TDD*, total daily dosage.

- **Notes**
    - This option is usually meant for patients using NPH as their basal insulin rather than a long-acting insulin analogue, as it is given twice daily; for some people, taking basal insulin in the morning may tide them over lunch.
    - TDD may be calculated as 0.2—0.3 units/kg to start.

Basal insulin
- If starting as a new regimen, initial dosage is ≤5 units bid if the person is lean or ≥10 units bid if the person is not lean.

- Alternatively, calculate the starting dosage as 50% TDD.
- Titrate the dosage of basal insulin according to the FPG and presupper blood glucose level by 1–2 units every 3 days until blood glucose level is at target.

Rapid-acting insulin

- Rapid-acting insulin dosage may be determined by the insulin/CHO ratio for breakfast and supper only in this regimen.
- Alternatively, rapid-acting insulin dosage may be determined as a "flat dosage" for each meal, based on average CHO intake for each meal, calculating at 1 unit/15 g CHO to begin.
- CF for rapid-acting insulin: 1–2 units for every 3.0 mmol/L >7.0 mmol/L at meals only; a CF dose is *not* recommended at night if the person is using a long-acting analogue, as this increases the risk for nocturnal hypoglycemia.

- **Premixed insulin: twice daily**

The use of premixed insulin is considered when optimal glycemic control is not sought and a more complex insulin regimen is impractical (Fig. 4.9).

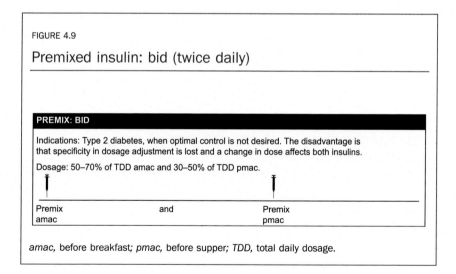

FIGURE 4.9

Premixed insulin: bid (twice daily)

PREMIX: BID

Indications: Type 2 diabetes, when optimal control is not desired. The disadvantage is that specificity in dosage adjustment is lost and a change in dose affects both insulins.

Dosage: 50–70% of TDD amac and 30–50% of TDD pmac.

| Premix amac | and | Premix pmac |

amac, before breakfast; *pmac,* before supper; *TDD,* total daily dosage.

Hypoglycemia management

Anyone using AHAs that can cause hypoglycemia or insulin needs to understand how to treat hypoglycemia.

Current evidence suggests that 15 g of glucose is required to produce an increase in blood glucose of 2.0 mmol/L within 20 minutes, with adequate symptom relief for most people who are experiencing an episode of hypoglycemia. When treating acute hypoglycemia, the following "rule of 15" is recommended.

Mild to moderate hypoglycemia (blood glucose 2.8—4.0 mmol/L)

1. Treat with *15 g* of rapid-acting CHO.
   - Examples of 15 g of CHO include the following:
     - Four chewable glucose or dextrose tablets (preferable), chew; although other fast-acting glucose preparations are available (glucose gel or liquid glucose), tablets are the most convenient and commonly used
     - $^3/_4$ cup (175 mL) fruit juice or regular soft drink
     - Six Life Savers (1 = 2.5 g CHO), chew
     - Table sugar (3 teaspoons/packets dissolved in water)
     - 1 tablespoon (15 mL) honey, swallow quickly to prevent coating the oral mucosa
2. Wait 15 minutes and re-treat if necessary
3. If the next meal is >1 hour away eat a snack containing 15 g CHO and a protein source, such as:
   - $^1/_2$ sandwich
   - Cheese and six to seven crackers

Severe hypoglycemia (blood glucose <2.8 mmol/L)

1. Treat with *20 g* of rapid-acting CHO
2. Recheck blood glucose in 15 minutes and re-treat with 15 g CHO if blood glucose is <4.0 mmol/L
3. If the next meal is >1 hour away, eat a snack containing 15 g CHO and a protein source
4. If individual is ≥10 years of age, an external caregiver can administer 1 mg glucagon subcutaneously or intranasally

Case studies
Marilyn

Marilyn is a 54-year-old woman who is new to your practice. She would like a diabetes assessment, as her sister was diagnosed with T2 diabetes recently. Marilyn describes herself as "relatively healthy," although she would like to lose the 9 kg that she has gained over the years. She has no significant medical history. Aside from her sister's recent diagnosis of diabetes, Marilyn also relates that her brother underwent coronary bypass surgery 4 years ago and is "doing quite well."

She does not smoke. Briefly, on examination, she is overweight with a body mass index (BMI) of 30 kg/m^2. Her blood pressure, sitting, is 140/88 mm Hg. The rest of her examination was unremarkable.

- **What is your approach?**

Marilyn has a number of risk factors to warrant screening her for diabetes: age, current BMI, and family history of diabetes and CVD in a first-degree relative. Marilyn can be screened in several ways. As she does not complain of any classical symptoms of diabetes, such as polydipsia, polyuria, blurred vision, or unexplained weight loss, performing a random blood glucose test (looking for a random plasma glucose >11.1 mmol/L) is not indicated.

Conventionally, she could have an FPG test (looking for FPG >7.0 mmol/L) or a more involved 75-g oral glucose tolerance test (OGTT) looking for a 2 hour value >11.1 mmol/L. Of note, the 2 hour value of 7.8—11.0 mmol/L would indicate prediabetes. Most easily, Marilyn can have a nonfasting glycated hemoglobin (A1C) test, looking for an A1C ≥6.5%. Also, of note, an A1C of 6.0%—6.4% would indicate prediabetes.

- **Marilyn's A1C result is 6.2%. What does this mean? What is your management plan?**

Marilyn's A1C of 6.2% indicates prediabetes. With prediabetes, Marilyn is at risk not only for T2 diabetes but also for CVD. With respect to her prediabetes, lifestyle changes are the first management strategy. A full assessment of Marilyn's eating and activity patterns should be done. A referral to a community-based DHC team for lifestyle education would certainly help. In the meantime, simple suggestions such as cutting out junk food and fast food, decreasing portion sizes, and walking at least 30 minutes/day can help get her started. Easy office tools such as the plate method or handy portion guide can be used to determine appropriate portion sizes. It would also be helpful to have a discussion regarding the practicalities of exercise: Does she have a treadmill/exercise bike that is collecting dust? Can she put it somewhere she will use it, such as in front of the television? Would she prefer to walk outside? Does she have somewhere secure to walk outside? Does she have a pair of properly fitted walking shoes?

The question of medication may come up. Insulin sensitizers such as metformin could be started; however, greater emphasis should be placed on helping Marilyn make lifestyle changes that she can sustain over the long term. As part of her assessment, it would be reasonable for Marilyn to have a fasting lipid profile done in view of her brother's history of CVD. Lifestyle changes may also help regarding her lipid levels. If her low-density lipoprotein cholesterol (LDL-C) level is >2.0 mmol/L, serious consideration should be given to starting a statin if lifestyle changes do not bring her LDL-C levels into target. (See Chronic Complications of Diabetes chapter.)

- **Marilyn's A1C result is 7.8%. What does this mean? What is your management plan?**

By diagnostic criteria, Marilyn has diabetes. It would be prudent to confirm the diagnosis by repeating the test on another day or by conducting an alternative test. This confirmation may be needed to assure Marilyn of the diagnosis.

All that has been said about lifestyle changes applies here. In this scenario, Marilyn may want to consider adding medication to her lifestyle regimen. The medication of first choice would be metformin. Other options with this A1C result could include a DPP-4 inhibitor, a GLP-1 receptor agonist, or an SGLT2 inhibitor. A sulfonylurea might be an option; however, at this point, it would be lower down on the list, as sulfonylureas carry a risk of hypoglycemia and possible weight gain. Her lifestyle changes need to be initiated now. If it is discovered that Marilyn has a major lifestyle issue that is significant and can be addressed directly (for example, if she describes drinking a large quantity of fruit juice or regular pop every day), then medication can be forestalled for a brief time to assess the effect of these major lifestyle changes. Marilyn may decide against any medication at this time and work with her lifestyle changes. This should be reassessed in a timely manner, likely after 2—3 months.

- **Marilyn's A1C result is 10.2%. What does this mean? What is your management plan?**

Not only does Marilyn have T2 diabetes, her A1C level is high enough to have a serious discussion about starting more than one AHA at this time. If there is a concern for possible metabolic decompensation, i.e., Marilyn is experiencing significant symptoms of hyperglycemia, including unexpected weight loss, then serious consideration should be given to starting insulin at the same time.

- **Marilyn's A1C result is 14.8%. What does this mean? What is your management plan?**

*This may be surprising, as Marilyn has no symptoms of diabetes; however, it is still quite possible that she has acclimated to the high blood sugar levels. With this result, confirmation of the diagnosis is required **only** if it can be determined that Marilyn will not suffer any metabolic decompensation in the meantime.*

With this degree of hyperglycemia, no delay in management should occur. Again, any obvious lifestyle issue that may affect this result must be addressed. However, medication should also be started in a timely fashion. Here, consideration should definitely be given to a combination of oral and/ or insulin therapy from the beginning in a more aggressive approach to her diabetes. Oral therapy combinations in addition to insulin could include metformin and a sulfonylurea, or metformin and a DPP-4 inhibitor. Serious consideration could also include metformin and a GLP-1 receptor agonist. In terms of insulin, basal insulin would most likely be added. With this degree of hyperglycemia, initial aggressive therapy can always be modified as improvement occurs. Naturally, a thorough assessment for any possible diabetes-related complications must also be done.

Beverly

Beverly is a 52-year-old lean woman who is complaining of an unexplained weight loss of 5.5 kg within the past 3 weeks. She has been experiencing increased urination, particularly at night. She has also noted "a dry mouth" recently. Beverly has a history of hypertension, which is well controlled on a thiazide diuretic. She has a family history of T2 diabetes, affecting her sister. In the office, a capillary blood glucose level is measured at 16.0 mmol/L.

- **What is your assessment and management plan?**

*Beverly most decidedly has diabetes. By presentation, it is most likely T2 diabetes despite the relatively short onset of marked symptoms but T1 diabetes also remains a possibility with the rapidity and severity of symptoms. Although Beverly needs a confirmatory diagnostic test, it would be prudent to test her antibody status (glutamic acid, islet cell, and insulin autoantibodies) to assess for the possibility of T1 diabetes. **Her management should not be delayed because of the severity of her symptoms and the possibility that her metabolic condition could deteriorate before the confirmatory test is done.***

With this degree of hyperglycemia, initial management should be fairly intensive, with the start of basal insulin. Also, with T2 diabetes still high on the differential diagnostic list, Beverly should likely also be started on combination oral AHA therapy, such as the insulin sensitizer metformin and an insulin secretagogue, likely gliclazide, to decrease the risk of hypoglycemia. An insulin secretagogue will act more quickly than an SGLT2 inhibitor. As Beverly is already symptomatic and verging on metabolic decompensation, an SGLT2 inhibitor would not be a good choice at this time, as it may also exacerbate metabolic decompensation through continued osmotic diuresis. With this degree of hyperglycemia, Beverly is at risk for decompensation, either hyperglycemic hyperosmolar nonketotic state or diabetic ketoacidosis.

At the same time, Beverly certainly requires a **priority** referral to a DHC team. In the meantime, some survival skills can be imparted. She can be taught SMBG by the diabetes education team on a priority basis or by a pharmacist. Simple lifestyle measures with respect to eating can also be taught in the office using the plate method or handy portion guide resources while waiting for more formal education, e.g., avoidance of any sugar-containing foods or beverages, such as fruit juice, regular soft drinks, sugary desserts, and snacks, as well as milk and fruit in large quantities.

Beverly obviously needs more aggressive management, which would mean initiation of insulin at this time. It is explained to Beverly that insulin is not a choice of "last resort." Rather, it is necessary to reverse the ongoing catabolic metabolism. The concept of basal/bolus insulin—with a long-acting basal insulin (glargine, detemir, degludec, or possibly NPH insulin bid) and the addition of rapid-acting insulin at meals—should be explained to Beverly and initiated.

Beverly asks if there are any other oral medication options. With her degree of hyperglycemia, adding other oral AHAs would likely be unsuccessful. With the addition of insulin, it would still be possible to add an SGLT2 inhibitor or a GLP-1 receptor agonist to provide further benefit later in her course.

Craig

Craig is a 50-year-old man with T2 diabetes, diagnosed 15 years ago. Ten years ago, he started insulin and stopped his oral medications, metformin and gliclazide, on the advice of another family physician. His current insulin regimen has remained the same and is as follows:

- NPH 16, Regular 6 before breakfast
- NPH 18, Regular 6 before supper

He monitors his blood glucose levels sporadically. He remembers that the last few values before meals (usually breakfast and supper) ranged from 10.0 to 14.0 mmol/L. The last A1C recorded is 12.0%. Yet, he describes nocturnal hypoglycemic episodes occurring two to three times/week. Upon further review, he recalls that his last eye examination was "a few years ago." He has begun to experience occasional erectile dysfunction, which has prompted him to ask about improving his diabetes control.

On examination, his blood pressure is 145/90 mm Hg. He has sensation to the 10-g Semmes-Weinstein monofilament test.

- **What further assessment is required?**

Craig needs a complete assessment of his diabetes, including glycemic control and complication assessment. His glycemic control is poor; the A1C of 12.0% reflects the 10.0–14.0 mmol/L glucose values before meals. He also needs a full complication assessment, including: a retinal examination; renal assessment with a urine albumin/creatinine ratio, eGFR, and serum creatinine; fasting lipid panel; and hormonal and penile vascular pressure investigations for his erectile dysfunction.

- **What management plan would you recommend?**

With this elevated A1C, a more intensive insulin regimen is recommended. Craig is not getting enough insulin and—understanding the pharmaco-kinetics of regular and NPH insulin—he likely has a mismatch of his insulin with his postmeal glucose rise. As well, his nocturnal hypoglycemia is likely due to the peak rise of his evening NPH insulin. Switching to a long-acting insulin analogue, such as glargine, detemir, or degludec, will rectify this issue. He would have a better match of insulin to food if he used rapid-acting insulin with meals. Craig needs to seriously consider changing to a basal/bolus insulin regimen. Working with a DHC team in the community will help him achieve this goal.

Other pharmacologic measures that may help Craig with his glycemic control include restarting metformin or adding an SGLT2 inhibitor or GLP-1 receptor agonist. A DPP-4 inhibitor may or may not be enough to help decrease his hyperglycemia.

Kim

Kim is a 36-year-old woman who presents at your office complaining of frequent vaginal yeast infections. She has tried various over-the-counter preparations with little success. It has been some time since Kim has been seen by you, her primary care provider. In the interim, it is noted that her weight has increased.

Currently her BMI is 34 kg/m^2. Kim denies any symptoms of diabetes. You ask Kim about diabetes-related risk factors. She states that her 72-year-old mother was recently diagnosed with T2 diabetes; no other family members have diabetes. Although her risk factor profile is modest, there is enough suspicion to screen Kim immediately in the office, if possible. A capillary glucose meter test in the office indicates her random blood glucose level is 13.0 mmol/L.

- **Does Kim have diabetes?**

The presentation of a typical acute hyperglycemia-related complication of a vaginal yeast infection in the presence of a capillary glucose of 13.0 mmol/L is enough to inform Kim of the diagnosis of diabetes and proceed with management strategies. For completeness, Kim should have a confirmatory A1C test.

- **What management approaches can be used here?**

An appropriate treatment for her symptomatic yeast infection is required. But without immediate management of her hyperglycemia, the treatment will likely fail. In this situation of an acute, albeit mild hyperglycemic complication, more aggressive therapy is required from the outset and can be modified later. Kim needs to receive key diabetes education with respect to lifestyle (i.e., nutritional intake, physical activity, and glucose monitoring) in a timely manner. As there is likely to be a delay before she can meet with a diabetes education team to discuss her eating patterns and to learn about SMBG, there are some simple strategies you can provide in the office. A quick 24-hour nutritional review will tell you if there are obvious changes required in her eating habits. Does she eat a lot of simple sources of sugar, such as regular soft drinks, fruit juices, fruit, or milk? Does she eat a lot of junk food or fast food? What is her approximate carbohydrate portion size at meals, i.e., how much bread, pasta, rice, or potatoes does she eat at a meal? Simply changing a few eating habits until she has a proper consultation with a dietitian can result in significant changes in her blood glucose control.

Learning about Kim's regular activity habits and introducing the concept of walking 20—30 minutes/day is also very useful; however, that advice will be part of the long-range plan. Right now, Kim needs fairly aggressive pharmacologic management. Metformin will be certainly useful to start, but it is unlikely to be sufficient if her random blood glucose level is 13.0 mmol/L. It will be helpful to add a more potent oral agent, such as a sulfonylurea or an SGLT2 inhibitor. Unfortunately, SGLT2 inhibitors may increase the risk of yeast infections, so this agent class should be considered later in Kim's course.

- **What would you do at this time?**

Kim is given a prescription for metformin and gliclazide MR. She is asked to start with low doses of both medications and titrate the dosages according to her tolerance and her blood sugar readings. A follow-up is arranged for 2 weeks' time. By then, she will have had a preliminary appointment with the community-based diabetes education team in her area. You also arrange an assessment for any long-term diabetes complications with the knowledge that Kim's T2 diabetes may have been present for some time prior to the diagnosis.

At follow-up, Kim reports that her yeast infection has resolved. With respect to her diabetes, she is presently taking metformin 1000 mg bid and gliclazide MR 60 mg od. Her blood glucose readings range from 5.0 to 9.0 mmol/L fasting and 6.0–12.0 mmol/L before her other meals.

- **What is your management plan?**

At this point, Kim may opt to continue titrating her gliclazide MR to 90 mg od, 120 mg being the maximum dose. Alternatively, she could add an SGLT2 inhibitor, a DPP-4 inhibitor, or a GLP-1 receptor agonist. A triple therapy approach would allow her to use combination therapy at submaximal dosages, thus decreasing the risk of adverse effects while maintaining sufficient therapeutic effect.

Brian

Brian is a 53-year-old man who has been struggling with his T2 diabetes for the past 10 years. He has been taking metformin 1000 mg bid and gliclazide 120 mg od for a number of years. Unfortunately, his weight has been climbing and his A1C remains elevated at 11.5%. He is discouraged and repeated discussions with the diabetes education team do not seem to help. His eating habits vary depending on his mood. His work is seasonal and as his work is labour-intensive, so is his physical activity. Outside of his daily work in season, Brian gets very little exercise. Fortunately, to date, assessment results for any long-term diabetes complications have been negative.

Recently, Brian received an unexpected "wake-up call." His 12-year-old son, Ryan, has started a track and field program at school with the goal of improving all students' fitness levels. Ryan wants his father to join him in some after-school runs. Brian starts.

- **What would you do at this time?**

An additional management option would be to add an SGLT2 inhibitor or a GLP-1 receptor agonist. Either will help lower Brian's blood sugar levels and promote weight loss.

Brian agrees to a trial of an SGLT2 inhibitor. Initially, he experiences urinary frequency but finds that he can adapt to this. At his return appointment after 2 months, he is happy to report that he has lost a modest amount of weight. Moreover, he has noticed that his blood sugar levels have improved, with a 1.5% decrease in A1C over the past 3 months.

- **What would you do at this time?**

In addition to maintaining his newfound exercise regimen, it is time for Brian to reassess his eating habits.

Andrea

Andrea is a 42-year-old woman who was diagnosed with T2 diabetes 2 years ago. At that time, she was significantly overweight. The diabetes diagnosis motivated her to seriously adjust her lifestyle habits. She consulted with the local DHC team, changed her eating habits, and started an exercise regimen. Over the past 2 years, she has brought her weight into a healthy range yet her A1C remains well over target at 9.5%.

- **What is your assessment and management plan?**

Andrea has successfully changed her lifestyle habits, a challenging undertaking for which she should be commended. The fact that her A1C is still high, and that her diabetes requires more involved management, is not her fault. This positive message must be conveyed to her.

Further reinforcement of her successful lifestyle changes should be done with her DHC team. Otherwise, Andrea could feel defeated and "stop trying, if it's not working." She needs to understand that she requires pharmacologic management, which will be more effective because of the solid base of lifestyle changes that she has made.

Options for pharmacologic management include metformin to begin. Andrea can be started on a low dose and instructed to titrate the dosage up slowly to avoid any adverse gastrointestinal effects.

Andrea returns after taking metformin for 2 months. Her current dose is 1000 mg bid. Yet, her A1C still remains above target at 9.0%. The addition of metformin has been effective, but only to a small degree.

- **What is your management plan?**

Andrea needs combination therapy. Options include an SGLT2 inhibitor, a medication from the incretin class (likely a DPP-4 inhibitor vs. a GLP-1 receptor agonist), or possibly an insulin secretagogue. The SGLT2 inhibitor will likely cause some weight loss and may improve her blood pressure because it effectively causes osmotic diuresis as it blocks renal reabsorption of glucose. The incretin acts to augment insulin's response while opposing the glycemic effect of glucagon. Consideration should be given to the choice of a DPP-4 inhibitor vs. a GLP-1 receptor agonist: the former is an oral agent, whereas the latter is injectable. The GLP-1 receptor agonist may be more effective, but it may also have greater gastrointestinal adverse effects, especially at the start of therapy. Andrea may feel more comfortable with an oral agent.

Choosing an insulin secretagogue, such as a sulfonylurea, is the common second choice. However, Andrea must be made aware that weight gain is likely with any sulfonylurea. After her successful weight loss efforts, this choice will likely not appeal to her. Also, in addition to her diabetes assessment, Andrea should be appropriately assessed for any diabetes complications.

Tony

Tony is a 19-year-old man who has been brought to your office by his mother. She, along with many other family members, has longstanding T2 diabetes. Now she is worried that Tony might be at risk. Tony is a husky young man, with a BMI of 28 kg/m^2. He has acanthosis nigricans in his neck folds, a clinical sign of possible insulin resistance, as do other members of his family. His blood pressure is 140/85 mm Hg.

- **How would you clinically assess Tony's risk for type 2 diabetes?**

Tony is at high risk for T2 diabetes: he has a strong family history of T2 diabetes and he has acanthosis nigricans, a risk factor for insulin resistance.

- **How would you further assess him?**

Tony should be screened in the usual fashion. He has no symptoms of hyperglycemia, so he should have an FPG, OGTT, or A1C performed. In this case, it would be better to opt for either of the two latter tests, as they will provide more information about possible impaired glucose tolerance, a form of prediabetes.

- **What is your management plan?**

Not only does Tony possibly have prediabetes or T2 diabetes, his blood pressure is 140/85 mm Hg. While not technically diagnostic for hypertension (unless he has diabetes), this level is high for a 19 year old. Clearly, his blood pressure should be monitored, but consideration should be given to further renal investigations. The most effective approach for Tony is lifestyle changes. However, it may be difficult to convince him to exercise regularly and eat healthy foods. Community resources and his family's support may be good allies here.

References

[1] Gerstein HC, Colhoun HM, Dagenais GR, et al., REWIND Trial Investigators. Design and baseline characteristics of participants in the researching cardiovascular events with a weekly incretin in diabetes (REWIND) trial on the cardiovascular effects of dulaglutide. Diabetes Obes Metabol 2018;20(1):42—9.

[2] Kristensen SL, Rørth R, Jhund PS, et al., Cardiovascular, mortality, and kidney outcomes with GLP-1 receptor agonists in patients with type 2 diabetes: A systematic review and meta-analysis of cardiovascular outcome trials. Lancet Diabetes Endocrinol 2019;7(10):776—85.

[3] Mann JFE, Ørsted DD, Brown-Frandsen K, et al., LEADER Steering Committee and Investigators. Liraglutide and renal outcomes in type 2 diabetes. N Engl J Med 2017;377(9):839—48.

[4] Marso SP, Daniels GH, Brown-Frandsen K, et al., Liraglutide and cardiovascular outcomes in type 2 diabetes. N Engl J Med 2016;375(4): 311—22.

[5] Zinman B, Wanner C, Lachin JM, et al., EMPA-REG OUTCOME Investigators. Empagliflozin, cardiovascular outcomes, and mortality in type 2 diabetes. N Engl J Med 2015;373(22):2117—28.

[6] Neal B, Perkovic V, Mahaffey KW, et al., CANVAS Program Collaborative Group. Canagliflozin and cardiovascular and renal events in type 2 diabetes. N Engl J Med 2017;377(7):644—57.

[7] Perkovic V, Jardine MJ, Neal B, et al., CREDENCE Trial Investigators. Canagliflozin and renal outcomes in type 2 diabetes and nephropathy. N Engl J Med June 13, 2019;380(24):2295—306.

[8] Wiviott SD, Raz I, Bonaca MP, et al., DECLARE—TIMI 58 Investigators. Dapagliflozin and cardiovascular outcomes in type 2 diabetes. N Engl J Med 2019;380(4):347—57.

[9] Zelniker TA, Wiviott SD, Raz I, et al., SGLT2 inhibitors for primary and secondary prevention of cardiovascular and renal outcomes in type 2 diabetes: A systematic review and meta-analysis of cardiovascular outcome trials. Lancet 2019;393(10166):31—9.

[10] Zhu J, Yu X, Zheng Y, et al. Association of glucose-lowering medications with cardiovascular outcomes: An umbrella review and evidence map. Lancet Diabetes Endocrinol 2020;8(3):192—205.

DIABETES AND TECHNOLOGY

Abstract

A plethora of technologic advances have occurred in the field of diabetes management. New forms of continuous glucose monitoring systems, insulin pumps, and automated options on insulin pumps are just a few of the advancements discussed in this chapter.

Keywords: Automode insulin pumps; Continuous glucose monitoring; Flash glucose monitoring; Insulin pumps.

Practical Diabetes Care for Healthcare Professionals
ISBN 978-0-12-820082-7
https://doi.org/10.1016/B978-0-12-820082-7.00005-1

Introduction

Technologic developments in diabetes move so quickly that it could almost be said that current technology is the "old" or "soon to be old" and the future will quickly be upon us. The future of diabetes technology includes a variety of continuous glucose monitoring (CGM) systems that connect with smartphones and watches, and subcutaneous insulin delivery systems (i.e., insulin pumps) that are increasingly sophisticated in their functions in introducing more autonomy, whereby insulin rates are determined and delivered dependent upon CGM sensor data independent of the user.

Self-monitoring of blood glucose

Self-monitoring of blood glucose (SMBG) provides useful educational feedback to people with diabetes. Understanding target blood glucose levels (fasting and premeal, 4.0–7.0 mmol/L; 2 hours postmeal, 5.0–8.0 mmol/L) can help people assess the effect of their diabetes medication regimen. Ideally, SMBG results should instruct patients where medication adjustments are needed. Patients are taught (and encouraged) to adjust antihyperglycemic medication and/or insulin dosages depending on the glucose patterns determined by their monitoring.

Blood glucose meters

Technology is constantly evolving to improve SMBG. Many blood glucose meters have functions that record the time and dosage of medication (especially insulin), record daily and weekly blood glucose averages, estimate A1C, and calculate insulin dosages according to a preset algorithm. They also have applications to record and upload blood glucose readings on personal or designated family or other individuals' smartphones, as well as upload information to offsite diabetes healthcare team members. Many glucose meters have separate monitoring strips to check for ketones in the event of an intercurrent illness, which increases the risk of diabetic ketoacidosis.

Continuous glucose monitoring

Subcutaneous glucose sensors that continuously measure interstitial fluid glucose values and store the data are constantly evolving. CGM systems either operate independently or in conjunction with an insulin pump, thus providing 24/7 glucose monitoring. Some insulin pumps require the simultaneous use of a CGM sensor to determine insulin delivery rates.

With rapid technologic advancements, many CGM systems have slimmer, smaller, and longer-lasting glucose sensors and more improved displays than ever before, as well as applications to link blood glucose data to smartphones and smart watches. They also allow uploading to provide different data reports, e.g., daily reports; weekly summaries; weekly, biweekly, and monthly glucose averages; and estimated A1C values. Many allow blood glucose targets to be set and will sound an alarm when those targets are exceeded. From a practical sense, most CGM systems are water resistant; some are waterproof.

Rather than measuring capillary blood as the typical glucose meter does, these sensors measure interstitial fluid glucose levels. There will be a lag between results from capillary and interstitial glucose values but often it is not significantly different. Some CGM systems require ongoing calibration with capillary glucose levels. Some of these systems can be affected by large dosages of acetaminophen or acetylsalicylic acid.

Flash glucose monitoring
Flash glucose monitoring refers to CGM devices that use a subcutaneous sensor, usually placed in the upper arm. Flash glucose monitoring systems are easy to use and often cost less than other CGM systems; hence, they are increasing in popularity. As with CGM systems, flash monitoring measures glucose levels on a separate handheld scanner or in some instances directly on a smart phone. Alternatively, results can be linked to smartphones and smart watches and uploaded to provide various data reports. As with other CGM systems, flash systems are water resistant, allowing users to shower and bathe while wearing them. They are almost considered waterproof, as they can take diving pressure up to 3 meters deep. The external scanner works through heavy clothing, even winter coats, which is a practical bonus.

Any of the newer technologies have limitations that must be explained to the user. Such limitations can include some degree of inaccuracy in the first 24 hours as the system equilibrates itself, sensor placement, and varying accuracy at either high or low glucose readings. With the use of flash glucose monitoring systems, glucose levels at the low or high end should be verified by a capillary glucose check. Some individuals react to the sensor adhesive or find that the sensor falls off easily. Manufacturers provide recommendations to address these issues.

Insulin pumps

Essentially, insulin pumps are sophisticated devices that deliver insulin subcutaneously 24/7. Rapid-acting insulin is delivered continuously either through tubing from the external pump through an infusion site (often located on the abdomen) or directly from the pump "pod" into the subcutaneous site without the need for tubing. In the former model, all monitoring and programming can be displayed and adjusted on the pump itself or, in some instances, on a smartphone. In the latter model, all monitoring and programming appears on a separate handheld device.

Most insulin pumps are still "open-loop" systems. This means that the person wearing the pump must program a set of basal insulin rates to run continuously in the background and program insulin/carbohydrate (CHO) ratios in order to set appropriate bolus dosages to be delivered when eating. The pumps allow users to program numerous basal rates and will calculate bolus dosages using various insulin/CHO algorithms once the amount of CHO is entered. The pumps also program insulin sensitivity factors, which determine individualized calculated correction dosages of insulin for elevated blood glucose levels. Targets can be programmed as well, with alarms for high or low blood glucose levels. Many pumps are linked to CGM devices or, at the very least, SMBG results from blood glucose meters can be linked to them. Considerable training is required to successfully operate an insulin pump. Such training is provided by professional pump trainers, many of whom are experienced diabetes educators.

As technology progresses, newer insulin pumps are smaller, slimmer, and easier to program than previous models. Semi-closed loop systems are now available. In a semi-closed loop pump, the linked CGM can autonomously vary the basal insulin rate; hence, set programmed basal rates are not required. In such systems, the concept of "time in range" (TIR) has emerged. TIR depends on set glucose targets and displays TIR or %TIR rather than blood glucose levels. Bolus dosages are still calculated dependent on preset insulin/CHO ratios.

The future of diabetes technology, with complete closed-loop pumps (sometimes referred to as an "artificial pancreas"), where both basal and bolus insulin dosages are autonomously determined by the pump, is close at hand. Prototypes are currently being studied.

CHRONIC COMPLICATIONS OF DIABETES: ASSESSMENT AND MANAGEMENT

Abstract

Diabetes management involves more than glycemic control. The overall aim in diabetes management is to prevent the onset or delay the progression of chronic complications. Chronic complications are classified as microvascular (retinopathy, nephropathy, and neuropathy) or macrovascular (cardiovascular [including diabetes-related dyslipidemia], peripheral vascular, and cerebrovascular) in nature. People with type 1 diabetes should be assessed regularly for complications ≥15 years of age and 5 years' duration of diabetes. People with type 2 diabetes should be assessed upon diagnosis, as there may be a lag time between the true time of onset and diagnosis. This chapter addresses appropriate screening and ongoing monitoring for these complications and the management strategies for them.

Keywords: Cardiovascular disease; Cerebrovascular disease; Dyslipidemia; Nephropathy; Neuropathy; Peripheral vascular disease; Retinopathy; Semmes-Weinstein monofilament.

Practical Diabetes Care for Healthcare Professionals
ISBN 978-0-12-820082-7
https://doi.org/10.1016/B978-0-12-820082-7.00006-3

As the long-term complications of diabetes include retinopathy, nephropathy, neuropathy, and cardiovascular, cerebrovascular, and peripheral vascular diseases, it is easy to conceptualize diabetes as a predominantly vascular disease. Overall vascular protection starts with some general approaches, including the all-important lifestyle changes and smoking cessation. Table 6.1 summarizes the approaches needed for micro- and macrovascular diabetes complications. Specific interventions are addressed in more detail in the following.

TABLE 6.1

Summary of interventions for micro- and macrovascular complications

Clinical factor	Target population	Interventions
Vascular protection	All people with diabetes	• Glycemic control • Lifestyle modifications • BP control • ACE/ARB medications • Lipid control • Smoking cessation • ECASA
Hypertension protection	All people with diabetes and hypertension (with or without nephropathy)	• Hypertension recommendations
Renal protection	All people with diabetes and nephropathy (with or without hypertension)	• Nephropathy recommendations and vascular protection

ACE, angiotensin-converting enzyme; ARB, angiotensin II receptor blocker; BP, blood pressure; ECASA, enteric-coated acetylsalicylic acid.

Microvascular complications
Retinopathy
People with type 1 (T1) diabetes should have a retinal assessment after age 15 years and 5 years' duration of diabetes. People with type 2 (T2) diabetes should have a retinal assessment at diagnosis, as it is recognized that the true onset of T2 diabetes may precede the diagnosis by some time. Screening for retinopathy should be performed by an experienced eye-care professional, either in person or through the interpretation of retinal photographs.

Optometrists are qualified by their standard training to perform regular retinal screening. In some rural or remote jurisdictions, screening may occur by itinerant trained technicians taking retinal photographs or through the performance of fundoscopy by trained healthcare professionals, e.g., nurses.

The follow-up interval for individuals with minimal or no retinopathy is every 1–2 years. Table 6.2 outlines screening guidelines for retinopathy.

TABLE 6.2

Screening for retinopathy

When to initiate screening

- For T1 diabetes, $\geq$15 years of age; screening annually after 5 years of diabetes
- For T2 diabetes, at time of diagnosis; screening thereafter as determined by the examiner, every 1–2 years

Screening methods

- 7-standard field, stereoscopic color fundus photography with interpretation by a trained reader (gold standard)
- Direct ophthalmoscopy or indirect slit lamp fundoscopy through dilated pupil
- Digital fundus photography

If retinopathy is present

- Establish appropriate monitoring intervals (1 year or less) with an eye-care specialist
- Maintain glycemic, BP, and lipid targets
- Screen for other diabetes complications

If retinopathy is not present

- Rescreen every 1–2 years
- Maintain glycemic, BP, and lipid targets
- Screen for other diabetes complications

BP, blood pressure; *T1*, type 1; *T2*, type 2.

Chronic kidney disease: nephropathy and hypertension

Screening for chronic kidney disease (CKD) in T1 diabetes should start at age 15 years, with annual screening occurring when diabetes has been present for 5 years. Screening for CKD in T2 diabetes should occur at the time of diagnosis and annually thereafter. CKD screening consists of a spot random urine albumin-to-creatinine ratio (uACR), as well as an estimated glomerular filtration rate (eGFR) and serum creatinine levels.

CKD in diabetes is diagnosed as follows: **random uACR >2.0 mg/mmol and/ or eGFR <60 mL/min/1.73 m^2 confirmed by repeat uACR >2.0 mg/mmol in 2 of 3 tests or repeat eGFR <60 mL/min/1.73 m^2, both within 3 months**.

The presence of confirmed microalbuminuria represents the earliest indication of nephropathy. Some laboratories quantify the uACR as microalbuminuria versus macroalbuminuria. Those patients with either micro- or macroalbuminuria can be considered to have nephropathy/CKD, unless another cause of albuminuria can be identified.

Interventions for microalbuminuria and nephropathy are outlined in Table 6.3, while follow-up therapies are outlined in Table 6.4.

TABLE 6.3

Interventions for nephropathy

Intervention	Considerations
Management of hypertension: this is the most important aspect of the intervention for nephropathy	• Hypertension in adults with diabetes should be treated to achieve a target BP <130/80 mm Hg
ACE inhibitor or ARB for kidney protective effect	• Serum creatinine and potassium levels checked at baseline and within 2 weeks of initiation or titration of therapy
Optimal glycemic control	• Reinforce physical activity, appropriate nutritional intake, and SMBG • Initiate or adjust medication, as necessary
Smoking cessation	• Smoking affects renal vasculature and hypertension
Assess lipids	• Microalbuminuria can be a marker for dyslipidemia
Antiplatelet therapy (ECASA)	• 81–325 mg/day is recommended for adults with additional CVD risk factors or for secondary prevention in those with CVD

ACE, angiotensin-converting enzyme; *ARB*, angiotensin II receptor blocker; *BP*, blood pressure; *CVD*, cardiovascular disease; *ECASA*, enteric-coated acetylsalicylic acid; *SMBG*, self-monitoring of blood glucose.

TABLE 6.4

Follow-up actions for nephropathy

Action	Considerations
Treat hypertension	• Target BP <130/80 mm Hg
Monitor renal function by eGFR or CrCl	• eGFR is generally used
Monitor ACE inhibitor/ ARB therapy	• Serum creatinine levels may rise to as much as 30% above baseline, stabilizing within 2–4 weeks • No upper limit of creatinine regarding contraindication, but caution should be exercised when CrCl <30 mL/min or eGFR <60 mL/min/1.73 m^2 • Serum potassium level, as it may rise • uACR after 3 months and annually, to assess reduction
Indications for referral	• uACR persistently >60 mg/mmol • eGFR <30 mL/min/1.73 m^2 • Serum creatinine level >30% above baseline within 3 months of ACE or ARB therapy • Inability to achieve target BP

ACE, angiotensin-converting enzyme; ARB, angiotensin II receptor blocker; BP, blood pressure; CrCl, creatinine clearance; eGFR, estimated glomerular filtration rate; uACR, urine albumin-to-creatinine ratio.

Emerging evidence now indicates that the glucagon-like peptide 1 (GLP-1) receptor agonist and sodium glucose co-transporter 2 (SGLT2) inhibitor classes of antihyperglycemic agents (AHAs) show reduction in adverse renal outcomes and can be considered renal protective. Consideration should be given to adding these classes of medication to the glycemic regimen, if appropriate [1–3].

Hypertension

Hypertension in adults with diabetes should be treated to achieve a target BP <130/80 mm Hg. Management includes lifestyle intervention as well as the initiation of antihypertensive therapies, listed in the following in the order of choice (combination therapy is often required):

- Angiotensin-converting enzyme (ACE) inhibitor/angiotensin II receptor blocker (ARB),

- Dihydropyridine calcium channel blocker,
- Thiazide diuretic.

Neuropathy

Diabetic neuropathy can affect the sensory, motor, or autonomic nervous systems. Classifications and descriptions of diabetic neuropathy are noted in Table 6.5.

TABLE 6.5

Classifications and descriptions of diabetic neuropathy

Classification	Description	Interventions
Diffuse symmetric polyneuropathy	• Common presentation is peripheral numbness and tingling, involving the hands and feet • Severe presentations have variable types of pain that cause sleep disruption • Neuropathic pain must be distinguished from intermittent claudication	Anticonvulsants[a] • Gabapentin • Pregabalin • Valproate Antidepressants[a] • Amitriptyline • Duloxetine • Venlafaxine • Opioid analgesics • Capsaicin cream • Topical nitrate spray
Focal mononeuropathies Cranial Peripheral Radiculopathy Diabetic amyotrophy	• e.g., Third nerve palsy with ptosis • e.g., Carpal tunnel syndrome, foot drop • Pain in truncal spinal nerve distribution • Proximal neuropathy manifested by pain, proximal muscle weakness, and muscle atrophy	• Usually resolves spontaneously • May respond to treatment for peripheral neuropathy

TABLE 6.5

Classifications and descriptions of diabetic neuropathy—cont'd

Classification	Description	Interventions
Autonomic neuropathy Gastrointestinal dysfunction	• Gastroparesis with vomiting, abdominal bloating, and pain	• Gastrointestinal motility pharmacotherapy, such as domperidone at a maximum dose of 10 mg tid with meals • Frequent small meals • Consider basal/bolus insulin regimen with rapid-acting insulin after meals as blood glucose starts to rise
	• Diarrhea	• Antidiarrheal medications
	• Constipation	• Increase water and dietary fiber intake
Genitourinary dysfunction	• Difficulty with micturition • Incontinence or incomplete emptying (neurogenic bladder) • Erectile dysfunction • Retrograde ejaculation	• Options for erectile dysfunction include phosphodiesterase type 5 inhibitors, vacuum pump, intrapenile prostaglandin injection, or prosthesis • Urology referral
Cardiovascular dysfunction	• Postural hypotension	• Compression stockings • Mineralocorticoid medication
	• Atypical angina	• High index of suspicion
Other	• Hypoglycemia unawareness	• Frequent SMBG
	• Anhidrosis, resulting in dry, cracked feet	• Moisturizers

SMBG, self-monitoring of blood glucose.
[a]Allow 6—8 weeks for effect.

Screening: use of a monofilament to detect neuropathy

The 10-g Semmes-Weinstein monofilament consists of a nylon filament mounted on a handle that has been standardized to deliver a 10-g force when applied properly. Screening with a monofilament is a validated method of assessing for the presence of peripheral neuropathy; it also helps the clinician to determine the risk of foot ulceration.

The monofilament should be applied to the dorsal and plantar surface of the great toe and the plantar aspects of the metatarsal heads (Fig. 6.1). The duration of time with which the monofilament should be in contact with the skin should be 2 seconds. Ideally, the application should occur twice at the same site. Avoid applying the monofilament to ulcer sites, calluses, scars, or necrotic tissue.

FIGURE 6.1

Semmes-Weinstein monofilament

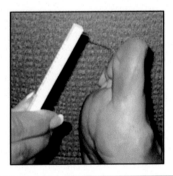

To perform a monofilament examination ask the patient to indicate when and where they can feel the monofilament touching their foot. Protective sensation is deemed to be present at each site if the patient correctly answers 2 of 3 applications.

Table 6.6 identifies risk categories and interventions using the Semmes-Weinstein monofilament.

Table 6.7 shows classifications and interventions for diabetic foot ulcers.

TABLE 6.6

Risk categories and interventions using the Semmes-Weinstein monofilament

Category	Classification	Interventions
0	• Intact protective sensation	• Low to no risk of foot complications • Education to be provided • Specialized footwear not necessary at this time • Examine feet at each visit or at least every 4—6 months
1	• Absent protective sensation • Normal foot morphology • No history of ulceration	• Examine feet at each visit or at least 4 times per year • Appropriately fitted footwear with a soft insole • Education to be provided
2	• Absent protective sensation • Foot deformity present • Plantar ulceration absent	• Examine feet at each visit or at least 4 times per year • Appropriately fitted footwear with a suitable insole • Education to be provided
3	• Absent protective sensation • History of plantar ulcer	• Examine feet at each visit or at least 4 times per year • Appropriately fitted footwear with a suitable insole (may need custom footwear) • Education to be provided

TABLE 6.7

Classification and interventions for diabetic foot ulcers

Wagner's grade	Criteria	Interventions
0	• Skin intact • No open lesions • May be nonblanching erythema	• Pare callus • Appropriate footwear to protect feet and reduce pressure over pressure points

Continued

TABLE 6.7

Classification and interventions for diabetic foot ulcers—cont'd

Wagner's grade	Criteria	Interventions
1	• Superficial skin ulceration (may be seen under area of high pressure)	• Pare callus to expose ulcer base; obtain specimen for culture if evidence of infection (i.e., redness, heat, pus) is present • A hydroactive gel covered by clean gauze is the simplest approach • Saline wet to dry dressings are an alternative if necrotic debris is present at the base of the wound • Pressure relief is critical for healing and can be accomplished with appropriate footwear, crutches, wheelchairs, and casting • Infected ulcers require antibiotics
2	• Deeper ulceration, associated with infection/cellulitis • Does not extend to bone	• Radiography to determine if bone is involved • Manage as for grade 1 ulcer; use antibiotics
3	• Ulcer has extended to deeper tissue layers such as bone • Has abscess formation or osteomyelitis	• Radiography to determine if bone is involved • Surgical debridement of infected bone • Appropriate antibiotics administered • Use noninvasive assessment of peripheral circulation (ankle brachial index); vascular surgical referral may be indicated

TABLE 6.7

Classification and interventions for diabetic foot ulcers—cont'd

Wagner's grade	Criteria	Interventions
4 (gangrene)	• Localized gangrene of toes, forefoot, heel	• Manage as for grade 3 ulcer • Urgent noninvasive assessment of peripheral circulation; vascular surgical referral may be indicated
5 (gangrene)	• Gangrene of entire foot	• Urgent assessment as for grade 4 lesions • Vascular surgical referral

Antibiotic therapy for foot infections

While first-line therapies for many foot infections include cloxacillin, cephalexin, clindamycin, amoxicillin/clavulanic acid, or doxycycline, the increasing prevalence of methicillin-resistant *Staphylococcus aureus* (MRSA) renders the consideration of an agent such as trimethoprim/ sulfamethoxazole an option in situations where the risk of MRSA-related infection is high. In patients who require intravenous antibiotic therapy, intravenous vancomycin is an appropriate first-line therapy for the management of infections caused by MRSA.

Although these antibiotic choices are suggested as empiric therapy, the ideal approach is to obtain a specimen for culture, initiate empiric therapy, and modify the therapy according to the results of the culture (Table 6.8).

TABLE 6.8

Interventions for foot complications

Complication	Intervention
• Nonblanching erythema over pressure points	• Reduce pressure with appropriate footwear
• Calluses and corns	• Reduce pressure with appropriate footwear • Pare carefully • Use pumice stone
• Cutaneous fungal infections • Intertrigo	• Clotrimazole cream 1% or tolnaftate cream 1% or powder applied twice daily • May require antibiotics for superimposed bacterial infection • Keep affected skin areas dry • Use antifungal cream
• Toenail abnormalities • Paronychia (nail bed infections)	• May be hypertrophic (thick and hornlike) • Cut nails every 3—6 weeks straight across to prevent formation of sharp edges • Twice-daily saline solution soaks and adequate nail care • Systemic antibiotics may be necessary
• Cellulitis	• Requires antibiotics; the route of administration (oral vs. parenteral) will depend on the severity of the infection
• Claw foot • Charcot foot	• Appropriate footwear and orthotic devices • For acute Charcot foot reduce deformity by removing pressure by immobilizing foot in cast • For established Charcot foot, appropriate insoles and shoes are required
• Ischemia • Intermittent claudication	• A painful, cold, and white extremity is a surgical emergency (may indicate acute occlusion) • Regular foot care and as much walking as possible to build collateral blood flow • Referral to a vascular surgeon

Macrovascular complications
Dyslipidemia

Diabetes is associated with a high risk of vascular disease (two- to four-fold greater than that of people without diabetes). Indeed, cardiovascular disease (CVD) is the primary cause of death among people with diabetes. Thus aggressive management of all cardiovascular risk factors, especially dyslipidemia, is very important. Table 6.9 identifies target lipid values for people with diabetes.

TABLE 6.9

Target lipid value based on level of risk

Risk level	LDL-C (mmol/L)
High (most patients with diabetes)	$\leq 2.0^a$

apo B, apolipoprotein B; *CVD*, cardiovascular disease; *HDL-C*, high-density lipoprotein cholesterol; *LDL-C*, low-density lipoprotein cholesterol; *TC*, total cholesterol.
[a]For individuals at high risk and who also have established CVD consider a target LDL-C <1.8 mmol/L; an alternative target is non-fasting apo B $\leq$0.8 g/L or non-HDL-C (TC minus HDL-C) <2.6 mmol/L.

Routine lipid screening should begin at age 40 years or earlier if diabetes has been present for >15 years and the patient is >30 years of age. The lipid profile is determined by a simple overnight fasting test and repeated annually if no abnormalities are identified or repeated every 3—6 months to check the effect of therapy. For those individuals in whom a prolonged fast is not feasible due to concerns regarding hypoglycemia stemming from their diabetes regimen, it is acceptable to measure nonfasting apolipoprotein B or non-high-density lipoprotein cholesterol (non HDL-C) (i.e., total cholesterol [TC] minus HDL-C) levels.

Table 6.10 addresses the treatment of dyslipidemia.

TABLE 6.10

Treatment of dyslipidemia

Lipid status	Therapy
LDL-C above target	Lifestyle modification plus statin[a,b]

LDL-C, low-density lipoprotein cholesterol.
[a]If a statin does not achieve target LDL-C, a second-line agent (e.g., cholesterol absorption inhibitor [ezetimibe], bile acid sequestrant [colesevelam, cholestyramine, colestipol], or PCSK9 inhibitor) may be added.
[b]If triglyceride level is >10.0 mmol/L, a fibrate may be used to reduce the risk of pancreatitis.

Cardiovascular disease
• Electrocardiographic (ECG) screening

For individuals with T1 or T2 diabetes, a baseline resting electrocardiography (ECG) should be performed, and repeated every 2 years, in the following situations:

- Age >40 years
- Diabetes duration >15 years and age >30 years
- End-organ damage (micro- or macrovascular)
- Cardiac risk factors

• Stress testing: indications

Following are the indications for a stress test. It is important to realize that in the presence of autonomic neuropathy, angina may present atypically, e.g., sharp chest pain, left arm/shoulder/jaw pain only, or shortness of breath only. Be aware of these atypical presentations in a patient with diabetes at risk for CVD.

- Typical or atypical cardiac symptoms (e.g., unexplained dyspnea, chest discomfort)
- Signs or symptoms of associated diseases:
  - Peripheral arterial disease,
  - Carotid bruits,
  - Transient ischemic attack,
  - Stroke,
  - Resting abnormalities on ECG.

• Management of cardiovascular disease

Beyond the essentials as summarized earlier with optimization of glycemic, lipid, and blood pressure control, as well as smoking cessation and healthy lifestyle adherence, emerging evidence indicates that certain classes of AHAs also provide long-term cardiovascular benefit. It is important to consider the addition of such medications in the individual at risk for or with documented CVD.

Emerging therapies for diabetes and cardiovascular disease

The SGLT2 inhibitor class carries the strongest evidence to reduce CVD outcomes. Major adverse cardiovascular events (MACE)—defined as a composite of total death, myocardial infarction, stroke, hospitalization for heart failure, and revascularization—are often the main outcome assessed in clinical trials. In clinical trials, the SGLT2 inhibitor empagliflozin reduced cardiovascular events, cardiovascular death, nonfatal myocardial infarction, or nonfatal stroke (i.e., a lower rate of a primary cardiovascular outcome and of death from any cause). Another SGLT2 inhibitor, canagliflozin, reduced cardiovascular death, nonfatal myocardial infarction, or nonfatal stroke. Neither of these outcomes are identified as MACE, but do assess major components of the MACE composite. A third SGLT2 inhibitor, dapagliflozin, while showing lesser evidence in reducing MACE, has been shown to reduce the incidence of hospitalization due to heart failure [4—6].

The GLP-1 receptor agonist class has also been shown to reduce CVD outcomes in clinical trials. Liraglutide reduced cardiovascular events, cardiovascular death, nonfatal myocardial infarction, and nonfatal stroke [7]. Emerging evidence indicates a cardioprotective benefit with semaglutide [7,8].

In fact, these two classes of medications, SGLT2 inhibitors and GLP-1 receptor agonists, are now considered vascular-protective. Consideration should be given to adding one or possibly both these classes of medications to the glycemic regimen, if appropriate. Ongoing studies will hopefully provide further evidence of possible CVD benefit from a wider and newer range of AHAs of these classes of medications.

Case study
Pat

Pat is a 56-year-old woman complaining of increased thirst and urination for the past 3 months. She has lost 4.5 kg unexpectedly but is happy about this weight loss because, as she tells you, "I have been trying to lose weight for years." She also tells you that years ago she was told she had "borderline diabetes" by a previous family doctor.

To date, Pat's medical problems have only included hypertension. Her medications include hydrochlorothiazide 25 mg od, calcium and vitamin D supplements, and a multivitamin supplement.

Pat has a sister with T2 diabetes and a brother who had a heart attack 3 years ago. She has never smoked.

On examination, her blood pressure, sitting, is 150/92 mm Hg. She appears tired but otherwise well. She is overweight, despite the recent 4.5 kg weight loss. Her BMI is 35 kg/m^2, placing her in the obese category.

- **What is your assessment and management plan?**

Pat has typical symptoms of diabetes: thirst, polyuria, unexpected weight loss, and fatigue. She has risk factors for diabetes, including age, obesity, and a family history. Moreover, Pat was told about "borderline diabetes" in the past. This very likely indicates that she had blood glucose levels diagnostic for diabetes previously, but somehow the message was not communicated properly.

Clinically, Pat has T2 diabetes. Still, confirmation is required. In the presence of these classical symptoms, a random plasma glucose ≥ 11.1 mmol/L is diagnostic for diabetes. From a practical perspective, many offices have glucose monitors available and an initial check of Pat's random glucose levels would be helpful.

Her random venous plasma glucose is 14.6 mmol/L.

- **What is your assessment?**

This is diagnostic for diabetes but should be further confirmed by means of a venous plasma test, most commonly an A1C $\geq 6.5\%$. Her A1C is 8.7%, again confirming the diagnosis of diabetes.

- **How long has she had diabetes?**

Pat has probably had diabetes for years. Likely, at the time she was told about "borderline" diabetes, she already had it. There is often a long lag period between true onset of T2 diabetes and diagnosis, which can be due to unawareness of or true lack of any symptoms associated with T2 diabetes.

- **What further assessment does she require?**

You have determined that Pat has T2 diabetes and has probably had it for quite some time. Therefore she may already have developed chronic complications of diabetes. Accordingly, Pat needs to be assessed for glycemic control and undergo a diabetes complication risk assessment as well.

Her clinical assessment should include a review of the symptoms of hyperglycemia, her usual eating and activity habits, and her understanding of and attitude toward diabetes. In terms of the complication assessment, this means a clinical review of any possible symptoms attributable to the presence of retinopathy, neuropathy, or nephropathy, as well as cardiovascular, peripheral, or cerebrovascular complications. One hint: Pat has hypertension. Often, hypertension can predict the presence of nephropathy. The laboratory investigations should include assessment for both glycemic control and long-term complications.

- **What is your management plan?**

Diabetes education is the fundamental first step for Pat. Find the community-based resource that can help Pat understand her diabetes and the effect that her eating and activity habits will have in managing her diabetes. Some simple office resources (see Glycemic Management chapter) can be employed until Pat can access further community-based education. Remember, behavior changes take time.

Pat's results indicate her A1C is 8.7%. With this A1C, although Pat may be making the necessary lifestyle changes to improve her diabetes, you should give serious consideration to starting medications now. The first-line choice, given her A1C, would be metformin, an insulin sensitizer.

Do not forget Pat's diabetes complication risk assessment. She needs:
- *Retinal eye screen by an experienced eye-care professional, most likely an optometrist;*
- *Nephropathy screen with a uACR and an evaluation of renal function with an eGFR and serum creatinine level assessment;*
- *Lipid profile;*
- *Monofilament assessment of her feet for protective sensation.*

Three months later, Pat returns for reassessment and reports the following self-monitoring of blood glucose results:
- Fasting, 7.0—9.0 mmol/L
- Before meals and at bedtime, 9.0—14.0 mmol/L

Her resting blood pressure is 150/90 mm Hg. Her repeat A1C is 8.5% and her uACR is 160 mg/mmol.

- **What would you do?**

Although improved, Pat's blood glucose values are still not in target. A review of her lifestyle will help. Adding another oral agent to metformin, such as a DPP-4 inhibitor or a GLP-1 receptor agonist, which will augment her insulin action and depress counterregulatory glucose rise, may help. Alternatively, adding an SGLT2 inhibitor may also help. The benefits and potential adverse effects of these classes of agents should be discussed with Pat before a decision is made.

If repeat blood pressure readings are >130/80 mm Hg and/or two out of three uACR results indicate nephropathy, Pat needs to start either an ACE inhibitor or ARB to decrease proteinuria and control blood pressure to <130/80 mm Hg.

Further review of Pat's laboratory results reveals that her fasting lipid profile is as follows:

- TC, 6.5 mmol/L
- Triglyceride, 5.8 mmol/L
- HDL-C, 0.95 mmol/L
- Low-density lipoprotein cholesterol (LDL-C), 4.3 mmol/L
- TC/HDL, 6.8 mmol/L

- **What would you do?**

Pat has an LDL-C that is well above the target of 2.0 mmol/L for people with diabetes. Initially, she should talk with the dietitian member of the diabetes healthcare team to find out where she can make changes in her diet that will help improve her lipid status. There are a number of nonpharmacologic strategies that may help. Certainly, she should also consider starting a statin. As her A1C improves, her triglyceride level will also improve. Once these measures have begun, her lipid status should be rechecked in 3 months.

Pat follows the dietary recommendations and is also prescribed an ACE inhibitor and a statin. You follow her every 3—4 months and her diabetes is stable, although her A1C remains above target at 8.5%. With her most recent assessment, Pat complains of "bloating." Further questioning reveals that she has early satiety, often accompanied by nausea, when she eats. There are days where she does not eat much and then finds her blood glucose levels drop, resulting in symptoms of hypoglycemia. She denies constipation or diarrhea.

- **What would you do?**

Clinically, Pat seems to be exhibiting typical symptoms of gastroparesis, an autonomic complication of her diabetes. Often, this complication is diagnosed clinically; sometimes a nuclear scan absorption test is used to confirm the diagnosis. In this test, a radioactive-labeled scrambled egg is eaten by the patient as a standard meal and the rate of digestion of the labeled egg can be tracked. Measures that can be used to help Pat include adding dietary fiber and water to her diet. Gastrointestinal motility medications, e.g., domperidone, can also be given at mealtimes. With this autonomic neuropathic complication identified, closer surveillance for any further sensory or autonomic neuropathies should be performed.

Going forward, Pat has been found to have diabetes-related microvascular complications of nephropathy and neuropathy, as well as a macrovascular-related complication of dyslipidemia. A complete assessment for the presence or progression of all micro- and macrovascular complications must be part of Pat's regular appointments. Naturally, attaining optimal blood glucose control will also help delay the progression of her complications.

References

[1] Mann JFE, Ørsted DD, Brown-Frandsen K, et al., LEADER Steering Committee and Investigators. Liraglutide and renal outcomes in type 2 diabetes. N Engl J Med 2017;377(9):839—48.

[2] Perkovic V, Jardine MJ, Neal B, et al., CREDENCE Trial Investigators. Canagliflozin and renal outcomes in type 2 diabetes and nephropathy. N Engl J Med June 13, 2019;380(24):2295—306.

[3] Mann JFE, Ørsted DD, Brown-Frandsen K, et al., LEADER Steering Committee and Investigators. Liraglutide and renal outcomes in type 2 diabetes. N Engl J Med 2017;377(9):839—48.

[4] Zinman B, Wanner C, Lachin JM, et al., EMPA-REG OUTCOME Investigators. Empagliflozin, cardiovascular outcomes, and mortality in type 2 diabetes. N Engl J Med 2015;373(22):2117—28.

[5] Neal B, Perkovic V, Mahaffey KW, et al., CANVAS Program Collaborative Group. Canagliflozin and cardiovascular and renal events in type 2 diabetes. N Engl J Med 2017;377(7):644—57.

[6] Wiviott SD, Raz I, Bonaca MP, et al., DECLARE—TIMI 58 Investigators. Dapagliflozin and cardiovascular outcomes in type 2 diabetes. N Engl J Med 2019;380(4):347—57.

[7]   Marso SP, Daniels GH, Brown-Frandsen K, et al., LEADER Steering Committee; LEADER Trial Investigators. Liraglutide and cardiovascular outcomes in type 2 diabetes. N Engl J Med 2016;375(4):311—22.

[8]   Marso SP, Bain SC, Consoli A, et al., SUSTAIN-6 Investigators. Semaglutide and cardiovascular outcomes in patients with type 2 diabetes. N Engl J Med 2016;375:1834—44.

ACUTE COMPLICATIONS OF DIABETES: ASSESSMENT AND MANAGEMENT

Abstract

Diabetic ketoacidosis (DKA) and hyperglycemic hyperosmolar nonketotic (HHNK) state are the two most serious acute complications of diabetes. They both carry a significant risk of morbidity and potential mortality. Although DKA is recognized readily in type 1 (T1) diabetes, it is often not appreciated that it can also occur in type 2 (T2) diabetes, often evolving from HHNK state. Indeed, these acute complications may be the first presentation of a new diagnosis of either T1 or T2 diabetes. In either situation, there may be precipitating factors that must be investigated and treated. The precipitating factors differ with respect to T1 and T2 diabetes. In T1 diabetes, DKA is most commonly due to the deliberate or accidental omission of insulin and other causes, including sepsis, need to be ruled out. In T2 diabetes, the HHNK state or HHNK state resulting in DKA are most often caused by an intervening event such as sepsis, myocardial infarction, organ ischemia, or stroke. Hypoglycemia is another acute complication of diabetes—often the most common acute complication—and must be managed appropriately. This chapter outlines a logical and methodical approach for the management of these acute complications.

Keywords: Dextrose/glucose tablets; Diabetic ketoacidosis; Hyperglycemic hyperosmolar nonketotic state; Hypoglycemia.

Practical Diabetes Care for Healthcare Professionals
ISBN 978-0-12-820082-7
https://doi.org/10.1016/B978-0-12-820082-7.00007-5

Diabetic ketoacidosis

Diabetic ketoacidosis (DKA) is a serious acute complication of diabetes. It is generally associated with type 1 (T1) diabetes and is often the first presentation of diabetes. Yet, DKA can also occur quite commonly in type 2 (T2) diabetes.

DKA carries considerable morbidity and, unfortunately, even mortality. As such, it must be recognized and treated promptly, and interventions, including education and management strategies, should be initiated to prevent recurrence.

Definition

Following are the criteria that define DKA:
- Blood glucose: $\geq$14.0 mmol/L
  - Caveats: where blood sugars may be lower but other diagnostic criteria are met
    - Partially treated DKA usually occurs when the patient appropriately attempts to treat acute hyperglycemia at home with extra insulin but, unfortunately, it evolves into DKA.
    - Rarely, sodium glucose co-transporter 2 (SGLT2) inhibitors may cause euglycemic DKA where other diagnostic criteria exist but blood glucose levels are lower than those expected for DKA.
- Arterial blood gas: pH <7.3; often a venous blood gas test is done instead.
- Ketones: present.
  - Serum: β-hydroxybutyric acid (β-OHB); some blood glucose meters also measure serum ketones
  - Urine: acetoacetic acid
- Serum bicarbonate (HCO_3) <15.0 mmol/L or CO_2 <23 mEq/L; often the anion gap (AG) is measured or calculated as well, looking for an increased AG.

The differential diagnosis includes the following:
- Mixed metabolic acidosis, which could be a combination of other causes of acidosis such as lactic acidosis from dehydration or organ (bowel) ischemia, acetylsalicylic acid-induced acidosis, methanol/ethylene glycol poisoning, renal disease, etc.
- Alcohol-related ketoacidosis.
- Hyperglycemic hyperosmolar nonketotic (HHNK) state, which is associated with T2 diabetes.

Causes

DKA is caused by an absolute or relative lack of insulin. In T1 diabetes, the most common cause is accidental or deliberate omission of insulin. DKA can be the first presentation of new-onset diabetes.

In those with known T1 diabetes, accidental omission of insulin usually results from undertreating an intercurrent illness with less, rather than more, insulin. With an intercurrent illness, there is usually an increased need for insulin related to stress responses/hormones, causing hyperglycemia.

There can also be situations where the omission of insulin is deliberate. Diabetes is a 24/7 job and patients sometimes get tired of it and want to take a "diabetes break." Other times, it may be acting out as a sign of frustration or anger. These causes should be explored once the DKA has resolved in order to employ the most appropriate interventions to prevent future occurrences.

In T2 diabetes, DKA is often precipitated by HHNK state. If the underlying cause of the HHNK state, such as acute illness, has not resolved, the metabolic derangement can evolve into DKA. In this situation, there is a need to thoroughly investigate any underlying precipitating causes, as they will need to be treated to allow the HHNK state/DKA to resolve.

Pathophysiology and clinical presentation

Generally, lack of insulin is the unifying pathophysiology that leads to all the metabolic problems in DKA. Lack of insulin leads to:

- *Increased lipolysis and AG-positive metabolic acidosis, i.e., ketoacidosis*: Simply put, lack of insulin decreases glucose transport into cells, calling for increasing sources of energy. This need will lead to a breakdown of hepatic glycogen, adding to hyperglycemia, then a breakdown of fat stores, releasing free fatty acids (FFAs). Ketone acids (also known as ketone bodies) are the breakdown product of FFAs, resulting in metabolic ketoacidosis. This metabolic acidosis is an AG-positive metabolic acidosis where the surplus anions originate from the ketone bodies. Hence the term diabetic ketoacidosis was coined. Metabolic ketoacidosis is the real cause of DKA morbidity. To compensate for the metabolic ketoacidosis, the body increases its respiratory rate in order to "blow off" CO_2 in response to the acidosis. This presents as Kussmaul breathing, the heavy labored breathing often seen in DKA. "Fruity" ketone breath can be detected as well.

- *Hyperglycemia*: Lack of insulin obviously leads to hyperglycemia and subsequent osmotic diuresis with polyuria. Continued osmotic diuresis will cause dehydration. With continued osmotic diuresis, excessive potassium (K^+) can be lost in the urine.
- *K^+ shifts*: Another compensatory mechanism the body has for metabolic acidosis is to shift acid (H^+) into the cells for K^+. Often, DKA will present with generous or even elevated K^+ levels for this reason. However, if the osmotic diuresis has been ongoing long enough, there may actually be a net K^+ loss. This needs to be recognized, as once insulin is started, K^+ will shift back into the cells as the acidosis is reversed. If net K^+ has been lost, then significant hypokalemia may occur.

Diabetic ketoacidosis management principles

- *Time course*: Generally, DKA requires 36–48 hours to resolve. A smooth steady resolution is desired to prevent any metabolic complications. In order to achieve this, maintaining a *clinical flowchart* to track laboratory values is key. Table 7.1 provides an example of such a flowchart.

TABLE 7.1

Clinical flowchart to track laboratory values in diabetic ketoacidosis

Time (hour)	BG	Na$^+$	K$^+$	CO$_2$	β-OHB	AG	IV fluids	Fluid addition	Insulin rate (U/hour)
0									
2									
3									
4									
6									
8									
12									
16									
20									

AG, anion gap; BG, blood gas; IV, intravenous; β-OHB, β-hydroxybutyric acid.

- *Metabolic ketoacidosis*: The first step in DKA management is the treatment of metabolic ketoacidosis. Insulin is used to stop the ongoing ketoacidosis, rather than to treat the hyperglycemia.
- *Dehydration*: Dehydration is caused by osmotic diuresis. Most patients require moderate intravenous (IV) fluid replacement, as detailed later.
- K^+ *shifts*: K^+ shifts into the cells as a compensatory mechanism for the metabolic acidosis. It is important to be aware of K^+ levels, as replacement may be needed early in the time course.
- *Hyperglycemia*: To prevent cerebral metabolic disequilibrium, hyperglycemia should be decreased at a slow, deliberate rate.

Some issues regarding DKA management remain controversial.

- *Fluid replacement—type and rate*: It is apparent that fluid deficits are not as extensive as once thought. The average fluid deficit is $\sim 3-6$ L (maximum) targeting replacement over 24–36 hours. To start, replacement will consist of 3–4 L over 12 hours. There are risks of fluid over-replacement; it is one of the contributing factors for the development of intracerebral edema, which is a devastating complication of DKA.
- *Rate of insulin infusion*: Another contributing factor to intracerebral edema or somewhat less ominously, cerebral disequilibrium, may be rapidly dropping blood glucose levels. Hence the insulin infusion rate should decrease hyperglycemia *no faster than 4–5 mmol/L per hour*.
- *When to give HCO_3*: There are many pitfalls in administering HCO_3, including:
  - Increasing hypokalemia,
  - Risk of paradoxical central nervous system (CNS) acidosis,
  - Shift of oxy-Hgb dissociation curve to left with decreased oxygen delivery to tissues,
  - Alkalosis favors ketone production in the liver.
- K^+ *replacement—KCL versus KPO$_4$*: There is little evidence to recommend K^+ replacement as KPO_4 in addition to or instead of KCL.

Diabetic ketoacidosis management

An initial clinical assessment should be made to determine if the patient is metabolically stable or unstable (with the latter requiring aggressive resuscitation). If relatively stable, then assess the degree of dehydration. Also assess for signs of sepsis or any other cause of DKA.

Initial laboratory investigations

Build the flowchart and send the required laboratory investigations.

Fluid replacement: type and rate

Most patients with DKA present with a moderate degree of dehydration (i.e., a fluid deficit of ~3—4 L); more severe dehydration may present with a fluid deficit of ~6 L. To prevent any potential complications from rapid or excessive fluid loading, fluid deficits (maximum 3—4 L) should be replaced over a period of 12 hours or longer. Normal saline (NS) is the usual fluid choice to be replaced by a dextrose-containing fluid once blood glucose levels have fallen to ~12.0—15.0 mmol/L. One example is listed in Table 7.2.

TABLE 7.2

Diabetic ketoacidosis protocol: fluid replacement

Fluid type	Time elapsed
NS 1 L	1—2 hours
NS 500 mL/hour × 2 (1 L)	3—4 hours
NS or D5W/1/2 NS 250 mL/hour × 8 (2 L)	~12 hours
Total: 4 L	

NS, normal saline.

Too rapid fluid replacement or over-replacement may contribute to the rare but significant complication of intracerebral edema.

Once blood glucose levels have reached ~12.0—15.0 mmol/L change NS to dextrose-containing fluid, i.e., D5W/1/2 NS.

Insulin administration

Regular insulin is generally used for the IV administration of insulin. Insulin is necessary to reverse ketoacidosis. Initial insulin infusion is usually started at 0.05 units/kg, which generally translates to ~2—4 units/hour. There is no need to administer a bolus dose at the start.

The aim is to decrease hyperglycemia by no faster than 4—5 mmol/L/ hour. Rapid decrease in blood glucose levels may lead to further metabolic derangement, such as CNS confusion, and possibly contribute to the development of intracerebral edema. Therefore insulin infusion should be **smoothly titrated by 1 unit/hour at a time** to achieve a steady decrease in blood glucose levels.

To prevent a relapse of DKA, the IV insulin infusion should continue until all evidence of ketones in the serum is absent (β-OHB <0.2 mmol/L). This process will take 36–48 hours.

K$^+$ replacement

Insulin will reverse the acidosis; as the acidosis reverses, K$^+$ will transfer back into cells, so note the original serum K$^+$ concentration to allow for replacement as needed.

Replace K$^+$ as follows:

K$^+$ ≥5.0	hold
K$^+$ 3.3–5.0	20 mmol/L
K$^+$ <3.3	40 mmol/L (hold insulin)
Maximum:	40 mmol/hour

There is no convincing evidence to suggest the use of KPO_4 rather than KCL.

HCO$_3$

Give HCO_3 only when pH <7.0.

Recognizing and avoiding pitfalls in diabetic ketoacidosis

It is important to acknowledge the following caveats to avoid pitfalls in DKA treatment:

- Avoid over-replacement of fluids
- Continue IV insulin until β-OHB <0.2 mmol/L
- Watch for hypokalemia
- Know when *not* to give HCO_3

Flowchart, flowchart, flowchart!

Keeping track of all the management parameters and the ongoing laboratory investigations will help make the resolution of DKA smooth and steady. It is very helpful to keep track of IV fluids hourly; glucose levels (usually through bedside capillary glucose monitoring), electrolytes, and AG every 2 hours; and β-OHB every 4 hours. These suggested time intervals can be adjusted as required.

With ongoing resolution of DKA, any precipitating causes (such as sepsis) should be treated. Preventive strategies should be reviewed for the future (refer to the section entitled "Sick day rules").

Case study
Josh

Josh is a 32-year-old man with T1 diabetes diagnosed when he was 17 years old. His usual insulin regimen is a basal/bolus regimen consisting of insulin aspart before meals utilizing an individualized insulin/CHO ratio of 1 unit/ 15 g CHO. He administers 25 units of glargine insulin at bedtime.

His most recent A1C, measured 3 months ago, was 7.8%. He is not known to have any diabetes complications.

Josh thought he was developing the "flu." He felt nauseated and stopped eating, although he kept drinking some fluids (water and plain broth). As he was not eating, he reduced his insulin dosage. Overnight, he developed worsening nausea and started vomiting. His blood glucose level on his meter started registering "HI." Accordingly, he went to the hospital.

In the ER, clinical assessment revealed that he complained of dizziness and nausea. He vomited once (clear fluid only). He denied fever, chills, digestive or urinary discomfort, and chest pain or discomfort but did admit to feeling short of breath. He looked unwell. He had the following signs of dehydration:

- Pulse, 110 bpm
- Blood pressure, 110/60 mm Hg lying and 95/50 mm Hg sitting
- Signs of metabolic acidosis:
  - Respiratory rate, 30 (i.e., Kussmaul breathing), ketotic breath
  - Glucose meter reading, "HI"

The clinical impression was most certainly DKA. Laboratory investigations were entered into a DKA flowchart (Table 7.3).

TABLE 7.3

Diabetic ketoacidosis flowchart

Time (h)	BG	Na^+	K^+	CO_2	β-OHB	AG	IV fluids	Fluid addition	Insulin rate (U/hour)
0	38.2	128	6.3	7.0	10.5	34	NS, 500 mL/hour		3

AG, anion gap; BG, blood gas; NS, normal saline; β-OHB, β-hydroxybutyric acid.

Josh was initially treated with IV NS at 500 cc/hour for 2 hours. An insulin infusion was started at 0.05 units/kg. Laboratory investigation included electrolytes, AG, β-OHB, and complete blood count. The flowchart depicted in Table 7.4 shows his progress throughout the ensuing 24 hours as the DKA protocol was followed, allowing him to recover. The only precipitating factor identified was his inadvertent omission of insulin when he was sick. Accordingly, sick day rules were reviewed with Josh before discharge.

TABLE 7.4

Diabetic ketoacidosis flowchart

Time (hour)	BG	Na$^+$	K$^+$	CO$_2$	β-OHB	AG	IV fluids	Fluid addition	Insulin rate (U/hour)
0	38.2	128.0	6.3	7.0	10.5	34.0	1 L NS		3
1	30.0						1 L NS		3
2	24.6	134.0	5.6	8.0	8.5	28.0	500 mL NS		3
3	20.5						500 mL NS		3
4	16.9	136.0	5.1	11.0	6.9	25.0	250 mL NS		3
6	14.3	135.0	4.9	12.0	4.0	20.0	250 ml D5W/1/2 NS		3
8	10.6	137.0	4.6	15.0	1.9	15.0	250 ml D5W/1/2 NS	K$^+$ at 20 mmol/L	2
12	12.9	136.0	4.5	17.0	1.3	14.0	250 ml D5W/1/2 NS	K$^+$ at 20 mmol/L	2
16	13.6	136.0	4.6	18.0	1.1	11.0	150 ml D5W 1/2 NS	K$^+$ at 20 mmol/L	3
20	10.3	136.0	4.5	22.0	0.8	9.0	150 ml D5W 1/2 NS	K$^+$ at 20 mmol/L	3

AG, anion gap; BG, blood gas; IV, intravenous; NS, normal saline; β-OHB, β-hydroxybutyric acid.

Hyperglycemic hyperosmolar nonketotic state

HHNK state is an acute hyperglycemic complication that is generally associated with T2 diabetes. As it occurs in older people either known to have T2 diabetes or who may have HHNK state as their initial presentation of diabetes, the process and presentation can be quite different from DKA.

Definition

As its name implies, HHNK state is a condition of hyperglycemia (usually quite significant hyperglycemia, higher than that seen in DKA) that is associated with significant dehydration (hyperosmolar) without any indication of DKA.

Pathophysiology and causes

By definition, people with T2 diabetes are not completely insulin deficient. T2 diabetes has the underlying pathophysiology of some level of insulin resistance and some degree of insulin deficiency. Therefore with an acute trigger causing metabolic derangement, there is still sufficient insulin to inhibit ketone production and subsequent ketoacidosis.

The list of possible precipitating causes of HHNK state is extensive. Common causes include infection/overt sepsis; acute vascular events, such as myocardial infarction or unstable angina with coronary insufficiency; acute peripheral vascular disease; acute gastrointestinal issues, such as bowel ischemia or bowel obstruction; pancreatitis; cholelithiasis; pulmonary embolus; or flulike syndromes. As there is most often a trigger, it is important to look diligently for that trigger because the metabolic derangement of HHNK state will not completely resolve until the underlying cause has been treated.

As people with T2 diabetes produce insulin, the acute trigger does not cause ketoacidosis. However, the acute situation will increase counter-regulatory stress hormone release, including catecholamines and cortisol, leading to hyperglycemia. Continued stress hormone hyperglycemia combined with insulin resistance and some degree of insulin deficiency lead to osmotic diuresis and dehydration. This process is subtle; patients do not feel as unwell as they would in the presence of DKA, so they do not seek medical attention as quickly. They often try to ameliorate the symptoms of increased thirst with sugar-containing fluids such as fruit juice or regular pop, especially if this is their first presentation with diabetes. Thus the dehydration progresses and by the time the patient seeks medical attention, they can have a profound metabolic derangement with significant hyperglycemia and dehydration. Protracted dehydration may also cause a degree of lactic acidosis. Rarely, the metabolic derangement is so prolonged and severe that the HHNK state can evolve into DKA. In this situation, it is often an AG-positive metabolic acidosis that is mixed, i.e., lactic and ketoacidosis.

As this process develops more slowly than DKA, and with an older population affected at presentation (often with underlying comorbidities), patients may be significantly more ill than younger patients who present with DKA.

Management principles

As with DKA, HHNK state requires a multifaceted approach, including administration of fluids and insulin, and treatment of any underlying precipitating causes. Similar to DKA, a clinical flowchart, particularly to track fluid replacement, is key (Table 7.5). The major issue of concern is

TABLE 7.5

Clinical flowchart to track laboratory values in the HHNK state

Time (hour)	BG	Na$^+$	K$^+$	CO$_2$	β-OHB	AG	IV fluids	Fluid addition	Insulin rate (U/hour)
0									
1									
2									
3									
4									
6									
8									
12									
16									
20									

AG, anion gap; BG, blood gas; HHNK, hyperglycemic hyperosmolar nonketotic; IV, intravenous; β-OHB, β-hydroxybutyric acid.

significant dehydration. The hyperglycemia will respond to fluid replacement; sometimes insulin is not required but if it is the dosage will be much lower than that used to treat DKA.

Management
• Fluid replacement

As patients with HHNK state are generally older and/or have comorbidities, attention must be paid to a slow reversal of the dehydration. Compared with DKA, rehydration will require less fluid at the beginning and more fluid over the long run, but at a slower rate. So, over time, these patients will actually receive a total of more fluid, but administered slowly!

• Rehydration

Average fluid loss is greater in HHNK state than in DKA, i.e., ~8–9 L that will be replaced over a number of days. The rate of fluid replacement should be tailored to the individual, but general guidelines are as follows:
   - 1 L NS ASAP
   - NS @ 500 mL/hour × 2 hours
   - NS @ 250 mL/hour × 4–8 hours depending on the response
   - NS @ 125 mL/hour (*less fluid, over a longer period*)
   - Follow electrolytes re: K^+

• Insulin

In the presence of HHNK state, insulin is administered to slowly and steadily lower blood glucose levels; it is not required to "turn off" ketogenesis. As opposed to DKA, insulin infusion is usually continued at a lower rate, e.g., 1–2 units/hour, not 0.05 units/kg as for DKA. Insulin administration may be temporary and may not be required once the HHNK state has resolved and other antihyperglycemic agents (AHAs) are started. As with all patients with T2 diabetes, lifestyle measures with or without AHAs often suffice.

Hyperglycemic hyperosmolar nonketotic state: recognizing and avoiding pitfalls
   - Determine precipitating factors
   - Avoid over-replacement of fluids
   - Administer lower, rather than higher, doses of insulin
   - Flowchart, flowchart, flowchart … especially to keep track of fluids

Case study
Helen

Helen is a 70-year-old woman who had been complaining of increasing thirst (i.e., "drinking everything and anything in sight") and fatigue over the past several weeks. She did not think she needed to see her primary care provider, as she thought she might have a cold or a virus.

One week later, she was found by her husband lying in bed, unable to get up. She was able to be roused but was drowsy and incoherent. In the ER, Helen was found to have a decreased level of consciousness. Her vital signs were as follows:

- Heart rate, 110 bpm
- Blood pressure, 125/75 mm Hg
- Temperature, 38.5°C

Investigations revealed the following:

- Blood glucose, 75.0 mmol/L
- Electrolytes, normal
- AG, 18 (mildly increased)
- β-OHB, 1.2 (mildly increased)
- Electrocardiogram, normal
- Chest X-ray, right lower lobe pneumonia

Helen was diagnosed with new-onset T2 diabetes, presenting with HHNK state secondary to pneumonia. She has no family history of diabetes and was never told that she had elevated blood glucose levels. The HHNK state was treated initially with IV NS as follows:

- 1 L NS ASAP
- NS @ 500 mL/hour × 2 hours
- NS @ 250 mL/hour × 8 hours
- NS @ 125 mL/hour

An insulin infusion was started at 1 unit/hour, coupled with dextrose at a low rate (75 cc/hour) to prevent unintentional hypoglycemia. Her pneumonia was treated with appropriate antibiotics. The hospital team kept track of her fluid balance by way of a flowchart. Her IV treatment with fluids and insulin continued for 4 days. Her blood glucose levels slowly decreased from 70.0 to 15.0 mmol/L during that time, after which Helen was able to eat full meals. She started oral AHAs and received in-hospital diabetes education and a referral for continued outpatient diabetes education after discharge and follow-up with her primary care provider.

Hypoglycemia

Hypoglycemia is often not thought to be an acute complication of diabetes. However, it is definitely the most common acute complication experienced by people with diabetes. Hypoglycemia can also be the most discomforting complication they will endure. Certainly it can lead to serious consequences, such as decreased consciousness or even loss of consciousness, seizures, personal accidents, or trauma. It can also result in the loss of a driver's license or even the loss of a job.

Recognition and treatment of hypoglycemia are among the survival skills taught to people newly diagnosed with diabetes. These skills are an absolute necessity for anyone taking an AHA that can cause hypoglycemia; the only exception is metformin. Table 7.6 classifies the severity of hypoglycemia and identifies the blood glucose levels for each.

TABLE 7.6

Hypoglycemia severity: symptoms and considerations

Severity	Symptoms and considerations	Blood glucose (mmol/L)
Mild	• Autonomic symptoms present • Individual is able to self-treat	<4.0
Moderate	• Autonomic and neuroglycopenic symptoms present • Individual is able to self-treat	2.8–4.0
Severe	• Usually requires the assistance of another person • Unconsciousness may occur	<2.8

Treatment of hypoglycemia

The "rule of 15" is the designation given to the approach to treat hypoglycemia.

• **Mild to moderate hypoglycemia (blood glucose 2.8–4.0 mmol/L)**

15/15 rule
1. Treat with 15 g of rapid-acting CHO.
   Examples of 15 g of CHO include the following:

- Four chewable glucose or dextrose tablets (preferable), chew; although other fast-acting glucose preparations are available (glucose gel or liquid glucose), tablets are the most convenient and commonly used
- $^3/_4$ cup (175 mL) fruit juice or regular soft drink
- Six Life Savers (15 g CHO), chew
- Table sugar (3 teaspoons/packets dissolved in water)
- One tablespoon (15 mL) honey, swallow quickly to prevent coating the oral mucosa
2. Wait 15 minutes and re-treat if necessary
3. If the next meal is >1 hour away, then eat a snack containing 15 g CHO and a protein source, such as
   - $^1/_2$ sandwich
   - Cheese and 6—7 crackers
- **Severe hypoglycemia (blood glucose <2.8 mmol/L)**
  - Treat with 20 g rapid-acting CHO in the form of chewable glucose or dextrose tablets (five tablets)
  - Recheck blood glucose level in 15 minutes and re-treat with 15 g CHO if blood glucose level is <4.0 mmol/L
  - If the next meal is >1 hour away, then eat a snack containing 15 g CHO and a protein source

If the person is unable to eat or swallow, 1 mg glucagon should be administered subcutaneously or intranasally by an external caregiver. Glucagon is as a counter-regulatory hormone that increases glucose levels. Glucagon will take 10—15 minutes to take effect.

Sick day rules
There are some general considerations patients can follow when they become ill that will prevent their diabetes from exacerbating their illness or prevent unintended complications from their diabetes medications.

- **Type 1 and type 2 diabetes: patients using insulin**
The key point to remember is that illness increases production of stress hormones, which in turn increases blood glucose levels. So although a patient may not feel like eating when sick, in fact, their blood glucose level may actually be higher rather than lower. In any event, increased glucose monitoring is necessary in addition to checking ketones (either urine or blood).

For elevated blood glucose levels, patients can take their "correction dose" of rapid-acting insulin (usually 1 unit for every 3 mmol/L blood glucose ≥7) every 4—6 hours to maintain blood glucose control. If blood glucose levels are elevated, the additional testing of ketones will inform patients whether they should add extra rapid-acting insulin to their "correction dose" to address the ketones, which is usually

- One extra unit of rapid-acting insulin for "small" ketones,
- Two for "moderate,"
- Three for "large."

It is also important for patients to ingest sugar-containing fluids on a regular basis, when their appetite is poor, to prevent hypoglycemia, e.g., $^1/_2$ cup of fruit juice or regular pop every 2—4 hours.

- **Type 1 and type 2 diabetes**

Fig. 7.1 is a useful mnemonic that identifies diabetes medications and other medications that should be stopped during illness, especially if there is a risk of dehydration. The medications on this list would also apply to those with T1 diabetes:

FIGURE 7.1

SADMANS

S	Sulfonylureas
A	ACE inhibitors
D	Diuretics, direct renin inhibitors
M	Metformin
A	ARB
N	Nonsteroidal anti-inflammatory agents
S	SGLT2 inhibitors

Source: Diabetes Canada 2018 Clinical Practice Guidelines for the Prevention and Management of Diabetes in Canada.
ACE, angiotensin-converting enzyme; ARB, angiotensin II receptor blocker; SGLT2, sodium glucose co-transporter 2.

DIABETES IN THE ELDERLY

Abstract

Management of diabetes in the elderly must take into consideration whether the older person is frail. Those who are frail need particular considerations to prevent acute diabetes complications, e.g., hypoglycemia and sepsis. In the elderly population the target A1C can be relaxed to ≤8.5%. Chronic diabetes complications or other chronic medical conditions may be the cause of significant comorbidities that complicate care. Chronic diabetes complications causing poor eyesight due to retinopathy, decreased renal function, poor balance and mobility due to neuropathy or stroke, or significant cardiovascular disease present individual management challenges. Medications, especially oral antihyperglycemic agents, may require dosage adjustment in the presence of comorbidities such as chronic kidney disease. Social circumstances may present a major challenge, i.e., if the elderly person is no longer independent and requires external caregivers for medication administration, blood glucose monitoring and even the daily necessities of meal preparation and hygiene.

Keywords: A1C targets; Blood glucose targets; Comorbidities; Frail elderly; Well elderly.

Practical Diabetes Care for Healthcare Professionals
ISBN 978-0-12-820082-7
https://doi.org/10.1016/B978-0-12-820082-7.00008-7

Introduction

The key concept in approaching diabetes in the elderly is to treat the whole person, not just their blood glucose. Often, this may be overlooked in a well-meaning attempt to achieve recommended blood glucose targets. Optimal diabetes management in the elderly must appreciate an individual's overall health, level of independence, and ability to manage multiple medications (for diabetes and coexisting conditions), as well as self-monitoring of blood glucose (SMBG), management of hypoglycemia, and possibly multiple insulin injections. Social circumstances may be of great importance for the elderly, i.e., the degree of support required for the person to manage their diabetes. Often, the risk/benefit ratio may favor "safer" blood glucose control over "target" blood glucose control. In fact, current recommendations suggest an optimal A1C range of 7.1%–8.5% for the elderly, particularly those with health challenges.

Approaching diabetes in the elderly requires some functional definitions. There are those who are the *well elderly* and those who are the *frail elderly*. Age is not the defining factor that distinguishes these two groups; rather, the definition is predicated upon the presence of comorbidities, which include microvascular complications (retinopathy, neuropathy, nephropathy) and macrovascular complications (cardiovascular, cerebrovascular, and peripheral vascular diseases) of diabetes. Comorbidities also include non-diabetes-related illnesses, which can contribute to an individual's frail state.

In the well elderly, glycemic targets are no different than those in other age groups. Although the risk of hypoglycemia exists for those who strive to maintain target blood glucose levels, this risk may have greater consequences in the elderly. Older people may be quite vulnerable to hypoglycemia and suffer from confusion, exacerbation of comorbid conditions (e.g., shortness of breath, angina), and falls. Thus the presence of comorbid conditions, as well as living circumstances, must be considered when determining appropriate glycemic targets in the elderly. Recommended blood glucose targets in the elderly are outlined in Table 8.1.

In elderly patients, clinical judgment should be used to determine if blood glucose targets should be relaxed. A safe blood glucose range can be determined, one that will reduce the risk of hypoglycemia. However, there remains a need to prevent persistent hyperglycemia that can lead to the occurrence of acute complications of hyperglycemia, namely, the increased risk of sepsis, hyperosmolar states, or possibly diabetic ketoacidosis. Also, the overall goal is to prevent the development and progression of long-term complications.

TABLE 8.1

Recommended blood glucose targets in the elderly

	A1C (%)	Preprandial blood glucose (mmol/L)	2-hour postprandial blood glucose (mmol/L)
Well elderly	<7.0	5.0–7.0	5.0–8.0/10.0
Frail elderly	<8.5	6.0–12.0	8.0–14.0

A1C, glycated hemoglobin.

Other considerations include the practicalities of administering diabetes medications (particularly insulin), especially in elderly patients who rely on external caregivers. In these situations, there may be limitations regarding when medications can be given, as well as issues with respect to access to food to prevent hypoglycemia and the ready availability of assistance by a caregiver.

The diabetes healthcare team

Oftentimes, the elderly require more support in order to manage their diabetes. In these circumstances, the diabetes healthcare (DHC) team expands to include a variety of allied healthcare professionals, including home care nurses, home care workers, and family members, who often play major caregiver roles.

Antihyperglycemic agents in the elderly

Essentially, the general recommendations and precautions regarding antihyperglycemic agents (AHAs) identified for the general diabetes population extend to the elderly population. However, there are some specific considerations for the elderly.

Metformin, an insulin sensitizer, remains a first-line oral agent; however, the clinician must remain aware of the relative and absolute contraindications regarding metformin and adverse effects may be more prevalent in the elderly. This class of medications needs to be dose-adjusted for renal function.

Sulfonylureas are still used commonly in the older population. However, glyburide may be associated with significant hypoglycemia. Thus priority should be given to gliclazide, as it carries less risk for hypoglycemia; also, gliclazide is available in a mono-release formulation, which aids in medication administration. Glimepiride is a long-lasting secretagogue that appears to have a lower risk of hypoglycemia than glyburide; it is also administered once daily.

The *incretin* class of medications, *glucagon-like peptide 1 (GLP-1) agonists* and *dipeptidyl peptidase-4 (DPP-4) inhibitors*, can be useful in the older population. However, concerns about the relationship between incretins and pancreatic inflammation or possible malignancies (pancreatic and medullary carcinoma of the thyroid) render a thorough medical review important before initiating therapy. It is also important to remember that, to date, no significant warnings have been reported for this medication class. Incretins, however, must be dose-adjusted for renal function.

Although *sodium glucose co-transporter 2 (SGLT2) inhibitors* can be useful, caution in the elderly is needed. This class of medication can cause significant dehydration resulting in low blood pressure, which could lead to light-headedness, syncope, and falls. This adverse effect can be exacerbated in the presence of other medications such as antihypertensive agents. Attention to maintaining hydration is recommended. Some classes of medications should be temporarily discontinued during an acute illness, and SGLT2 inhibitors certainly are in this category along with sulfonylureas and metformin. Rarely, euglycemic diabetic ketoacidosis may occur, particularly when this class of medication is not stopped during times of intercurrent illnesses.

Other drug classes, including *meglitinides* (short-acting insulin secre-tagogues) and *α1-glucosidase inhibitors*, have been used successfully in the elderly population. No specific concerns regarding these agents have been reported to date, aside from the usual concerns regarding hypoglycemia and gastrointestinal tolerance, in the case of α1-glucosidase inhibitors.

Renal function and antihyperglycemic agents
A number of diabetes medications require dosage adjustment in the presence of decreased renal function. Fig. 8.1 identifies dosage adjustment for estimated glomerular filtration rate (eGFR) for all classes of diabetes medications, including insulin. Many elderly patients may have decreased renal function as a result of increasing age alone and/or secondary to an underlying renal disorder, e.g., chronic kidney disease (CKD) as a complication of diabetes.

FIGURE 8.1

Antihyperglycemic agents and dosage adjustment for renal function

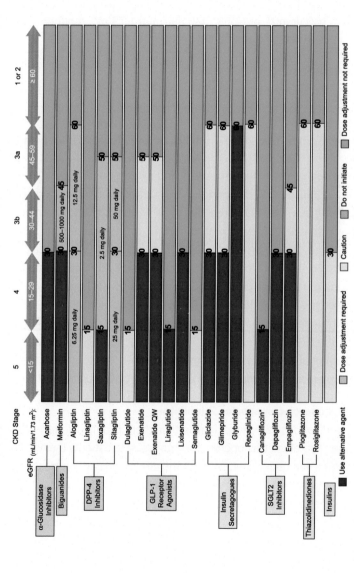

Source: Diabetes Canada 2018 Clinical Practice Guidelines for the Prevention and Management of Diabetes in Canada.
CKD, chronic kidney disease; CVD, cardiovascular disease; DPP-4, dipeptidyl peptidase-4; eGFR, estimated glomerular filtration rate; GLP-1, glucagon-like peptide 1; SGLT2, sodium glucose co-transporter 2.

Metformin

Renal function must be assessed before recommending metformin. In the presence of reduced renal function (defined as serum creatinine >130 μmol/L or eGFR <60 mL/min/1.73 m^2), metformin should be kept to a maximum dose of 500 mg bid. In the presence of worsening renal function with a serum creatinine >160 μmol/L or eGFR <30 mL/min/1.73 m^2, metformin should not be administered.

Sulfonylureas

There is evidence of a higher risk of hypoglycemia with decreasing renal function, so monitoring is required when prescribing sulfonylureas.

Incretins: dipeptidyl peptidase-4 inhibitors and glucagon-like peptide 1 agonists

People with decreased renal function, as indicated by serum creatinine >130 μmol/L (eGFR <60 mL/min/1.73 m^2), should be prescribed sitagliptin and saxagliptin at a dose that is reduced by 50%. Sitagliptin dose can be further reduced with an eGFR of 15–30 mL/min/1.73 m^2. Linagliptin and saxagliptin can be dose-reduced for eGFRs of 30 or 15 mL/min/1.73 m^2 for saxagliptin and 15 mL/min/1.73 m^2 for linagliptin, respectively. GLP-1 agonists can be kept at the usual dosages until the eGFR reaches 15–30 mL/min/1.73 m^2, depending on the formulation; liraglutide can be used until an eGFR of 15 mL/min/1.73 m^2 is reached; and exenatide/exenatide QW and lixisenatide can be used until an eGFR of 30 mL/min/1.73 m^2 is reached. For the newest GLP-1 agonist, semaglutide, experience in those with CKD is still limited; therefore caution is suggested in patients with an eFGR of <30 mL/min/1.73 m^2.

Sodium glucose co-transporter 2 inhibitors

As these medications can cause dehydration, there is a risk of prerenal acute kidney injury. Therefore it is important to emphasize to patients the need to keep well hydrated when taking them. As with the other medications, dosage adjustment should be made with decreasing renal function. Canagliflozin, empagliflozin, and dapagliflozin can all be used at the usual dosages for eGFR of 45 mL/min/1.73 m^2. Recent research shows that some of these medications can be used at a lower eGFR than previously indicated (Fig. 8.1). Although these agents can be used at lower eGFRs, caution should be used in the elderly.

Antihyperglycemic agents and acute illness

While precautions should be taken with certain AHAs in the presence of an acute illness, greater attention should be paid in the case of the elderly, as they may be significantly more vulnerable to potential adverse effects. SADMANS (Fig. 8.2) is a useful mnemonic that identifies diabetes medications and other medications that should be stopped when ill, especially if there is a risk of dehydration. Consideration should be made to temporarily discontinue their use until the individual has recovered and it is deemed safe to continue. The diabetes-related medications on the list would also apply to those with type 1 diabetes.

FIGURE 8.2

SADMANS

S	Sulfonylureas
A	ACE inhibitors
D	Diuretics, direct renin inhibitors
M	Metformin
A	ARB
N	Nonsteroidal anti-inflammatory agents
S	SGLT2 inhibitors

Source: Diabetes Canada 2018 Clinical Practice Guidelines for the Prevention and Management of Diabetes in Canada.
ACE, angiotensin-converting enzyme; ARB, angiotensin II receptor blocker; SGLT2, sodium glucose co-transporter 2.

Antihyperglycemic agent combinations in the elderly

Similar to younger adults with diabetes, there are a number of effective AHA combinations possible as long as the appropriate precautions are taken for the older population. One of the most common combinations includes an insulin sensitizer (metformin) plus an insulin secretagogue. Considering the reduced risk of hypoglycemia with gliclazide and, to a somewhat lesser extent, glimepiride, these agents would be the preferred secretagogues for use in elderly patients. With the advent of newer AHA classes, incretins (either DPP-4 inhibitors or GLP-1 agonists) or SGLT2 inhibitors in combination with metformin and/or gliclazide can be effective.

Many older people use weekly pill dispensers that they or their caregivers fill and maintain. Pharmacies commonly dispense oral medications in blister or bubble packs, which can be very helpful in maintaining medication adherence.

Insulin use in the elderly

Insulin can be very useful in managing diabetes in the elderly. An approach similar to the younger adult population is used, such as combinations of longer-acting insulins with AHAs, and progression to rapid- and long-acting insulin regimens as indicated. The long-acting basal insulin analogues glargine, detemir, and degludec have a lower risk of hypoglycemia than NPH insulin.

What follows is a practical guide to AHA and/or insulin regimens. The regimens considered to be most practical in the older person include the following:

- Addition of a basal insulin at bedtime while continuing the AHA regimen during the day.
- Use of basal insulin, NPH, or detemir twice daily, while continuing the AHA regimen during the day.
- Use of a premixed insulin regimen can be helpful, particularly for the elderly person who is reliant on external caregivers.
- Often, rapid-acting insulin can be used as a correction factor (CF) dosage at mealtimes when blood glucose levels are out of target.

Some older people prefer and successfully manage a more complex basal/bolus insulin regimen without issue. Where external caregivers are required, a more practical approach is needed. A fixed dosage of rapid-acting insulin can be given at each meal, with or without a CF added for either high, or, more importantly, to subtract insulin for low premeal glucose levels, along with basal insulin at bedtime. Also, use of a premixed insulin, particularly rapid and longer-acting premixes (Humalog Mix 25 or NovoMix 70/30).

Following is a short description of some insulin regimens that can be easily adapted to the older person with diabetes. If the situation calls for a more complicated basal/bolus insulin regimen, a practical approach or compromise can be found; usually, this consists of a predetermined "flat dose" of rapid-acting insulin with meals, as opposed to carbohydrate (CHO) counting, to calculate the dose of rapid-acting insulin each time.

Insulin/antihyperglycemic agent combinations

The insulin regimens outlined in the following are listed in the order in which they are commonly administered in type 2 diabetes, with particular reference to the elderly. However, any regimen may be chosen, depending on individual circumstances.

- **Bedtime insulin and antihyperglycemic agents**

This is a relatively simple method to introduce insulin into a combination regimen with oral agents (Fig. 8.3). Here, basal insulin is added at bedtime to help counteract hepatic glucose output during the night and thus lower fasting blood glucose in the morning. Starting the day with a lower fasting blood glucose level will allow the oral agents taken during the day to be more effective. NPH or one of the long-acting analogue insulins can be started as the bedtime basal insulin.

FIGURE 8.3

Bedtime insulin and AHAs

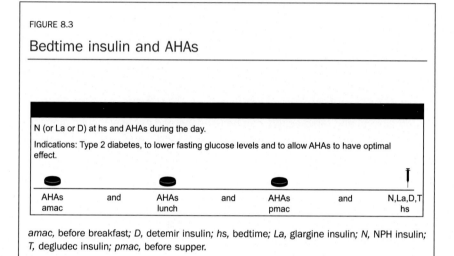

N (or La or D) at hs and AHAs during the day.

Indications: Type 2 diabetes, to lower fasting glucose levels and to allow AHAs to have optimal effect.

| AHAs amac | and | AHAs lunch | and | AHAs pmac | and | N,La,D,T hs |

amac, before breakfast; *D*, detemir insulin; *hs*, bedtime; *La*, glargine insulin; *N*, NPH insulin; *T*, degludec insulin; *pmac*, before supper.

- **Notes**
  - Start with ≤5 units hs if the person is lean; 8–10 units hs if the person is not lean.
  - Alternatively, calculate the starting dosage by 0.2–0.3 units/kg.
  - Titrate the dosage according to the first morning SMBG by 1–2 units every 3 days until the fasting plasma glucose (FPG) is at target.
  - Rapid insulin CF: 1–2 units for every 3.0 mmol/L >7.0 mmol/L can be used at meals, along with AHAs.

- **Daytime insulin and antihyperglycemic agents**

Once- or twice-daily basal insulin can be used with most oral agents during the day in effective combinations (Fig. 8.4). NPH is usually tried first in this regimen. Glargine or degludec is primarily used once per day, and detemir

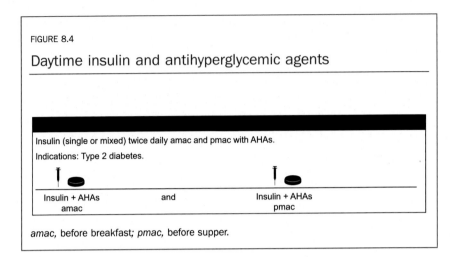

Daytime insulin and antihyperglycemic agents

Insulin (single or mixed) twice daily amac and pmac with AHAs.

Indications: Type 2 diabetes.

Insulin + AHAs   and   Insulin + AHAs
     amac   pmac

amac, before breakfast; *pmac*, before supper.

can often be used twice per day. Sometimes, a mixed insulin regimen, including basal and rapid-acting, can be used instead of basal insulin alone. In this case, the AHA would be metformin, glimepiride (which has an indication for use with daytime insulin), or possibly one of the incretin or SGLT2 inhibitor classes of agents.

- **Notes**
  - Long-acting analogue or intermediate-acting insulin.
  - Initial dosage: $\leq$5 units bid if the person is lean; $\geq$8–10 units bid if the person is not lean.
  - Alternatively, calculate the starting dosage by 0.2–0.3 units/kg.
  - Titrate the dosage according to SMBG, FPG, and presupper blood glucose by 1–2 units every 3 days until blood glucose is at target. Total daily dose of insulin may be split as either 67%/33% or 50%/50%.

- **Premixed insulin, twice daily**
- **Notes**
  - This regimen is intended for situations where a realistic compromise between optimal and safe blood glucose targets is required. The nature of premixed insulins renders it impossible to adjust one insulin in the mix without the other. This regimen may also offer a practical solution for a person who requires an external caregiver to administer the insulin.
  - When choosing a premixed insulin, it may be preferable to choose one of the rapid/basal options such as Humalog Mix 25 or NovoLog

Premixed insulin, twice daily

Indications: Type 2 diabetes, when optimal control is not desired and for those with difficulty differentiating insulins. The disadvantage is that specificity in dosage adjustment is lost and a change in dose affects both insulins.

Dosage: 50–70% of TDD amac and 30–50% of TDD pmac.

| Premix amac | and | Premix pmac |

amac, before breakfast; *pmac,* before supper; *TDD,* total daily dose.

Mix 70/30. The rapid insulin component matches the timing of food digestion and may result in smoother blood glucose control with a lower risk of hypoglycemia a number of hours after insulin and the meal (Fig. 8.5).

- **Basal/bolus insulin, four times daily**

I prefer the term "basal/bolus" for this regimen, as I believe it is a functional term that describes precisely the insulin regimen. It also more closely patterns physiologic insulin secretion (Fig. 8.6).

- **Notes**
  - Total daily dose (TDD) should be calculated as indicated in the following for basal and bolus insulin. Generally, the TDD is 50% basal and 50% bolus insulin.
  - Alternatively, TDD can be calculated as 0.2–0.3 units/kg to start.
  - Lastly, this regimen may be a stepwise progression from a previous insulin regimen, whereby previous insulin dosages can be adapted.

Basal insulin
  - If starting as a new regimen, initial dosage is ≤5 units bid if the person is lean and 8–10 units bid if the person is not lean.

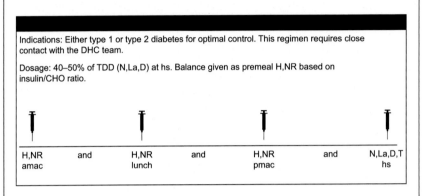

FIGURE 8.6

Basal/bolus insulin, four times daily

Indications: Either type 1 or type 2 diabetes for optimal control. This regimen requires close contact with the DHC team.

Dosage: 40–50% of TDD (N,La,D) at hs. Balance given as premeal H,NR based on insulin/CHO ratio.

| H,NR | and | H,NR | and | H,NR | and | N,La,D,T |
| amac | | lunch | | pmac | | hs |

amac, before breakfast; *CHO,* carbohydrate; *D,* detemir insulin; *DHC,* diabetes healthcare; *H,* lispro insulin; *hs,* bedtime; *La,* glargine insulin; *N,* NPH insulin; *T,* degludec insulin; *NR,* insulin aspart; *pmac,* before supper; *TDD,* total daily dose.

- Alternatively, calculate the starting dosage by using 50% of calculated TDD.
- Titrate the dosage of basal insulin according to the FPG by 1–2 units every 3 days until the FPG is at target.

Bolus insulin

- Rapid-acting insulin dosage may be determined by the insulin/CHO ratio, starting with 1 unit insulin/15 g CHO.
- Alternatively, rapid-acting insulin dosage may be determined as a "flat dosage" for each meal, based on an average CHO intake for each meal, calculating 1 unit/15 g CHO to begin. Alternatively the remaining 50% TDD may simply be distributed among the daily meals.
- Rapid-acting insulin CF: 1–2 units/3.0 mmol/L >7.0 mmol/L at meals only. A correction dose is not recommended at night if the person is using a long-acting analogue, as this increases the risk for nocturnal hypoglycemia.

- **Basal/bolus insulin, three times daily**

This is an alternative regimen that may help patients who have difficulty fitting in the lunchtime bolus insulin dose. It works better with NPH insulin to provide insulin coverage through lunchtime (Fig. 8.7).

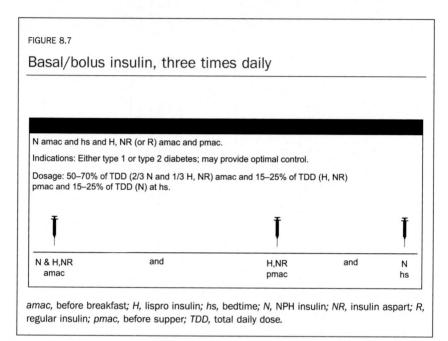

FIGURE 8.7

Basal/bolus insulin, three times daily

N amac and hs and H, NR (or R) amac and pmac.

Indications: Either type 1 or type 2 diabetes; may provide optimal control.

Dosage: 50–70% of TDD (2/3 N and 1/3 H, NR) amac and 15–25% of TDD (H, NR) pmac and 15–25% of TDD (N) at hs.

| N & H,NR amac | and | H,NR pmac | and | N hs |

amac, before breakfast; *H,* lispro insulin; *hs,* bedtime; *N,* NPH insulin; *NR,* insulin aspart; *R,* regular insulin; *pmac,* before supper; *TDD,* total daily dose.

- **Notes**
  - This option is meant for patients using NPH as their basal insulin rather than a long-acting insulin analogue.
  - TDD may be calculated as 0.2–0.3 units/kg to start.

Basal insulin
  - If starting as a new regimen, then for the basal insulin, initial dosage is ≤5 units bid if the person is lean and 8–10 units bid if the person is not lean.
  - Alternatively, calculate the starting dosage as 50% TDD.
  - Titrate the dosage of basal insulin according to the FPG and presupper blood glucose level by 1–2 units every 3 days until the blood glucose is at target.

Bolus insulin

- Rapid-acting insulin dosage may be determined by the insulin/CHO ratio for breakfast and supper only in this regimen.
- Rapid-acting insulin dosage may be determined as a "flat dosage" for each meal, based on average CHO intake for each meal calculating at 1 unit/15 g CHO to begin. Or, the remaining 50% TDD can be distributed among the daily meals.
- Rapid-acting insulin CF: 1–2 units/3.0 mmol/L >7.0 mmol/L at meals only and not at night if the person is using a long-acting analogue.

Hypoglycemia management

Anyone using AHAs that can cause hypoglycemia or insulin needs to understand how to treat hypoglycemia.

Current evidence suggests that 15 g of glucose is required to produce an increase in blood glucose level of 2.0 mmol/L within 20 minutes, with adequate symptom relief for most people who are experiencing an episode of hypoglycemia. When treating acute hypoglycemia, the following "rule of 15" is recommended.

Mild to moderate hypoglycemia (blood glucose 2.8–4.0 mmol/L)

1. Treat with 15 g of rapid-acting CHO
Examples of 15 g of CHO include the following:
   - Four chewable glucose or dextrose tablets (preferable), chew; although other fast-acting glucose preparations are available (glucose gel or liquid glucose), tablets are the most convenient and commonly used
   - $^3/_4$ cup (175 mL) fruit juice or regular soft drink
   - Six Life Savers (1 = 2.5 g CHO), chew
   - Table sugar (3 teaspoons/packets dissolved in water)
   - One tablespoon (15 mL) honey, swallow quickly to prevent coating the oral mucosa
2. Wait 15 minutes and re-treat if necessary
3. If the next meal is >1 hour away, then eat a snack containing 15 g CHO and a protein source, such as:
   - $^1/_2$ sandwich
   - Cheese and 6 to 7 crackers

Severe hypoglycemia (blood glucose <2.8 mmol/L)

1. Treat with 20 g of rapid-acting CHO
2. Recheck blood glucose in 15 minutes and re-treat with 15 g CHO if blood glucose level is <4.0 mmol/L
3. If the next meal is >1 hour away, then eat a snack containing 15 g CHO and a protein source
4. If individual is ≥10 years of age, an external caregiver can administer 1 mg glucagon subcutaneously or intranasally

Diabetes complications in the elderly

The basic approach to screening and intervention for both micro- and macrovascular complications is no different in the older person than in the general diabetes population. However, there are some specific issues that should be considered.

Retinopathy

Older people may already have vision issues (e.g., cataracts, glaucoma, or macular degeneration). In the presence of any of these eye conditions, monitoring for diabetic retinopathy on a regular basis by an experienced eye care professional takes on renewed importance, as visual deterioration from any cause presents a barrier to independent living.

Nephropathy

Hypertension, usually seen with nephropathy, can be challenging to manage in the elderly. While the choice of medications is no different than that in younger people with diabetes (i.e., angiotensin-converting enzyme [ACE] inhibitors or angiotensin II receptor blockers [ARBs]), there may be an increased risk of adverse effects such as postural hypotension leading to dizziness, difficulty in coping, and falls. These classes of antihypertensive medications can also increase potassium and creatinine levels. Older people may also have an increased prevalence of underlying CKD from another cause, which may exacerbate these recognized side effects of ACE inhibitors and ARBs and render the management of hypertension difficult. There may be a need to monitor renal function (serum creatinine levels and eGFR) and electrolytes more frequently.

Older people with marked CKD face many challenges with respect to dialysis. Indeed, much supportive care will be required for patients, whether they are undergoing hemodialysis or peritoneal dialysis.

Neuropathy, peripheral vascular disease, and foot care

The presence of the common peripheral sensory neuropathy can impair an older person's ability to mobilize safely. This can increase the risk of falls, particularly in those who may already have problems with balance or strength from another cause.

Peripheral vascular disease may have a higher prevalence in the elderly, especially in those with a history of smoking. Regular clinical assessment and a routine ultrasound screen of arterial brachial indexes are needed in these higher-risk individuals.

Foot care presents a major issue in the elderly population with diabetes. Regular foot assessment and care, including nail trimming, often requires support from external caregivers. If a person's foot becomes compromised by infection or ulceration, the necessary immobility required for healing can lead to further health problems.

Cardiovascular and cerebrovascular diseases

Cardiovascular disease and cerebrovascular disease are serious complications that require a complex management plan, including vascular assessment, and interventions such as angiography, angioplasty, or surgery. Recovery can be slow in the presence of comorbidities related to age and/or diabetes. Blood glucose control is of significant concern and requires close monitoring and medication adjustment. Often, in the acute situation, insulin presents the better choice for glycemic control; in the event that insulin is initiated, it is essential that the DHC team and caregivers monitor frequently for hypoglycemia and hyperglycemia.

Quality of life

Last, and certainly not least, is remembering the importance of quality of life. Blood glucose control should never be ignored; however, there is a need to revisit blood glucose targets regularly. The elderly, particularly the frail elderly, should have safe glycemic targets that ensure maintained good health but do not reduce quality of life.

Case study
Eileen

This case vignette is offered here to highlight many of the issues facing an elderly person with diabetes with the intent of increasing healthcare professionals' awareness regarding these issues and how they can be managed.

• Introduction

Eileen is an 86-year-old woman who was diagnosed with type 2 diabetes 25 years ago. For many years, her diabetes was controlled with the use of gliclazide 60 mg bid. She had her diabetes regularly assessed by her family doctor and she was told the disease was stable, with A1C ranging from 7.8% to 8.3%. Eileen is very conscientious about her diabetes: she monitors her blood glucose two or three times per day, usually before meals, and is very concerned if it exceeds 8.0–9.0 mmol/L.

• Surgery and hospitalization

However, Eileen has vascular disease, a complication of her diabetes, and she was hospitalized recently for vascular surgery. Unfortunately, the surgery was unsuccessful and she underwent a below-the-knee amputation to her left leg. This has changed her life dramatically. Prior to the amputation she was independent; currently, she is confined to a wheelchair. Once she is released from hospital, she must move into an assisted-living facility where meals are provided.

During her hospitalization, Eileen's blood glucose levels have risen and are no longer controlled by her previous medication. This was to be expected, given her inactivity during hospitalization and the counter-regulatory stress rise postoperatively. Her blood glucose levels range between 12.0 and 18.0 mmol/L before meals. This distresses Eileen, and this stress has made her blood glucose levels increase even further. Rapid insulin has been administered before meals, using a "sliding scale" approach. When Eileen was ready for discharge the insulin was stopped and she was placed back on gliclazide 60 mg bid.

• How does this situation affect Eileen's diabetes?

Prior to her hospitalization and surgery, Eileen was diligent in her diabetes management by eating balanced meals and monitoring her blood glucose levels frequently. Now, however, she feels that she has lost control of her life. She is no longer mobile and independent, and in the assisted-living facility, she will have little choice in her meals.

Now, in the assisted-living facility, the loss of control regarding her diabetes has only served to increase Eileen's anxiety and stress levels, which results in the unwanted effect of further increased blood glucose levels. Indeed, Eileen has noticed that her blood glucose levels regularly range between 12.0 and 22.0 mmol/L before meals. Her anxiety about her blood glucose levels is escalating, and the staff find that Eileen is becoming increasingly anxious. She refuses to eat because she is afraid of elevating her blood glucose levels even further; as a result, she has begun to experience low blood glucose levels, a combined effect of reduced nutritional intake and the continuation of gliclazide. Both Eileen and her caregivers are becoming increasingly frustrated. Eileen wants good blood glucose control again and the staff cannot understand why her blood glucose levels are "swinging" from high to low.

- **How could this situation have been addressed to improve the outcome?**

Eileen's concerns about her diabetes control need to be acknowledged. However, she must also be made aware that, for her situation, blood glucose control can be relaxed from the standard of 5.0–7.0 mmol/L before meals. A premeal range of 6.0–12.0 mmol/L and/or a 2-hour postmeal range of 8.0–14.0 mmol/L will protect Eileen from the acute complications of hyperglycemia. As Eileen is not frail, these target blood glucose targets will apply to her.

The maximum dose of gliclazide is clearly no longer adequate. Indeed, with her blood glucose levels so high, the addition of other oral medications will be unlikely to help the situation. Eileen needs insulin, but how can that be managed in her new situation?

There are a few strategies that might work. First, establishing a new, relaxed target blood glucose range. Second, it is important to communicate to Eileen and the staff caring for her. Adding basal insulin, NPH bid, or glargine, detemir, or degludec daily at supper or bedtime (a supper regimen may protect Eileen from any possible nocturnal hypoglycemia) along with an AHA during the day may work.

If this strategy still does not reduce Eileen's blood glucose levels to the new target range, then premixed insulin should be considered, rather than potentially confusing Eileen with a basal/bolus regimen. Choosing a premix of rapid- and longer-acting insulin would make more sense than a regular/ longer-acting premix to better time the rapid-insulin peak to the postmeal glucose peak. Using a basal or a premix bid would also help the staff if they will be administering the insulin, if Eileen is incapable of doing so.

The choice of an insulin/AHA combination or regularly scheduled insulin alone is a more proactive approach that will result in smoother blood glucose control, rather than simply using an insulin sliding scale.

- **Considerations**

    1. *Eileen's past experience of independent management of her diabetes and her continuing desire to remain independent in this practice.*
    2. *Deteriorating health problems that necessitate hospitalization, her diabetes control worsens, and many changes are made to her diabetes management.*
    3. *Eileen's increased anxiety and stress will only increase her blood glucose levels. Increased frustration on the part of her healthcare providers will also have the same effect.*
    4. *The staff would benefit from understanding that every time Eileen refuses to eat as a method of controlling her blood glucose levels, her blood glucose level will drop too low because the gliclazide is continued. This drop results in rebound hyperglycemia, and thus the cycle of hyperglycemia/hypoglycemia continues.*
    5. *Understanding on the part of staff can lessen Eileen's anxiety and help normalize her blood glucose control.*

PREGNANCY AND DIABETES

Abstract

Diabetes in pregnancy carries specific risks for both the baby and mother. Diabetes in pregnancy, either pre-existing diabetes or gestational diabetes mellitus (GDM), defines new blood glucose targets and glucose monitoring parameters to be followed throughout the pregnancy. GDM is diabetes that is first diagnosed during the course of the pregnancy. All pregnant women should be screened by 26–28 weeks' gestation, as this is when insulin resistance normally arises. Often GDM is managed with lifestyle changes. If target blood glucose levels are not met in a timely fashion, the current management recommendation is a basal/bolus insulin regimen. All women with GDM should undergo a 75-g oral glucose tolerance test between 6 weeks and 6 months postpartum to ensure that the GDM has resolved. Pre-existing diabetes carries its own specific risks for pregnancy. Preconception planning is recommended to ensure optimal glycemic control in order to prevent the risk of congenital anomalies. Appropriate assessment for identified chronic complications is also required, as these could worsen during the pregnancy. Diabetes in pregnancy is generally considered to be a higher risk pregnancy and requires close monitoring by both the diabetes and obstetric teams throughout.

Keywords: Gestational diabetes mellitus; Gestational diabetes screening; Postpartum diabetes screening; Preconception planning; Pre-existing diabetes.

Practical Diabetes Care for Healthcare Professionals
ISBN 978-0-12-820082-7
https://doi.org/10.1016/B978-0-12-820082-7.00009-9

Gestational diabetes mellitus

As with type 2 (T2) diabetes, the incidence of gestational diabetes mellitus (GDM) is increasing. It is important to recognize and manage GDM appropriately, as it is now understood that GDM not only increases the risk for future development of T2 diabetes in the mother but also increases the risk of early childhood obesity and possible early-onset T2 diabetes in the child.

GDM is defined as glucose intolerance with first onset or recognition during pregnancy. Risk factors for GDM include the following:

- Maternal age $\geq$35 years
- Family history of T2 diabetes
- Member of a high-risk ethnic group, including Indigenous, Hispanic, Asian, South Asian, and African populations
- Previous GDM
- Prepregnancy overweight/obesity
- Excess weight gain in current pregnancy
- Polycystic ovary syndrome
- Acanthosis nigricans (as associated with insulin resistance)
- Previous delivery of a large infant (>4.0 kg)

Many of these risk factors resemble those for T2 diabetes, as the pathophysiology of GDM is similar, with insulin resistance being the major factor. GDM typically occurs in the latter half of the second trimester, around 26–28 weeks' gestation. In all pregnancies, it is thought that increased insulin resistance arises from placental hormone secretion, including placental lactogen, cortisol, and estrogen, among others. In certain populations of pregnant women, particularly those with risk factors, this late second trimester insulin resistance cannot be overcome, resulting in the development of GDM.

Screening for gestational diabetes mellitus: two-step screening

All pregnant women should be screened for GDM at 24–28 weeks' gestation. If a risk factor, as described earlier, is identified earlier in the pregnancy, screening should be performed at that time. If the screen result is negative but the risk factor persists, screening should be repeated as per current recommendations. Earlier screening will identify those women with overt/pre-existing diabetes in whom the diagnosis had not yet been made.

The preferred screening test is a 50-g oral glucose load, administered at any time of day regardless of food intake, followed by a plasma glucose test at 1 hour:

- If the 1-hour value is $\geq$7.8 mmol/L, then proceed to the diagnostic 2 hour 75-g oral glucose tolerance test (OGTT).
- If the 1-hour value is $\geq$11.1 mmol/L, a diagnosis of GDM can be made.

Diagnosis of gestational diabetes mellitus

Table 9.1 depicts the 2 hour 75-g OGTT threshold values for diagnosis. If ≥ 1 values are met or exceeded, the diagnosis of GDM is made.

TABLE 9.1

2 hour 75-g oral glucose tolerance test threshold values for the diagnosis of gestational diabetes mellitus

Parameter	Blood glucose (mmol/L)
Fasting	≥ 5.3
1 hour	≥ 10.6
2 hour	≥ 9.0

Screening for gestational diabetes mellitus: one-step screening

An alternative diagnostic test, known as the one-step test, precludes the 1-hour, post-50-g screen; rather, it utilizes a 2 hour 75-g OGTT but has lower recommended threshold values. Table 9.2 outlines the parameters and blood glucose levels regarding the one-step test. One abnormal value is needed for diagnosis. Most centers, however, still utilize the two-step method.

TABLE 9.2

One-step test for diagnosis of gestational diabetes mellitus

Parameter	Blood glucose (mmol/L)
Fasting	≥ 5.1
1 hour	≥ 10.0
2 hour	≥ 8.5

Management of gestational diabetes mellitus

Nutritional therapy is the primary treatment for GDM. A woman diagnosed with GDM should be assessed and followed as required by the diabetes healthcare team to ensure that her nutritional intake is appropriate to achieve recommended glycemic control, appropriate weight gain, and adequate nutritional intake for both her and her baby. Accordingly, the dietitian is an important member of the team.

Prior to meeting with a dietitian, primary care providers can offer some practical tips that a patient can use in the meantime. Often, the distribution of carbohydrate throughout the day can make a real difference. Use the 24-hour recall method to determine where and how much carbohydrate is being consumed: Is breakfast all carbohydrate, with cereal, toast, milk, and/or juice being consumed? Does she eat significant quantities of carbohydrate-rich foods, such as rice, breads, bagels, potatoes, pasta, and baked goods? Fruits (especially grapes and melons), fruit juice, regular pop, and even milk are all considered carbohydrate-rich. Having her eat a balance of all food groups at each meal—utilizing either the plate method or the handy portion guide to ensure proper portion size—is a good start (Figs. 9.1 and 9.2).

FIGURE 9.1

Plate method to determine portion size

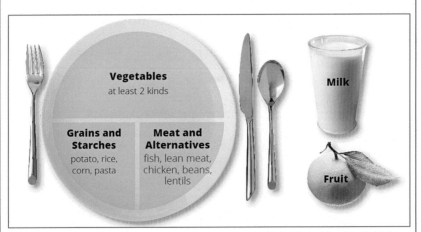

Source: Reproduced with permission from Diabetes Canada 2018 Clinical Practice Guidelines for the Prevention and Management of Diabetes in Canada.

FIGURE 9.2

Handy portion guide to determine portion size

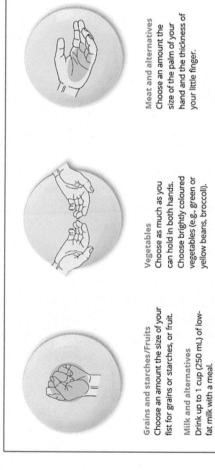

Grains and starches/Fruits
Choose an amount the size of your fist for grains or starches, or fruit.

Milk and alternatives
Drink up to 1 cup (250 mL) of low-fat milk with a meal.

Vegetables
Choose as much as you can hold in both hands. Choose brightly coloured vegetables (e.g., green or yellow beans, broccoli).

Meat and alternatives
Choose an amount the size of the palm of your hand and the thickness of your little finger.

Fat
Limit fat to an amount the size of the tip of your thumb.

Source: Reproduced with permission from Diabetes Canada 2018 Clinical Practice Guidelines for the Prevention and Management of Diabetes in Canada.

Physical activity should be encouraged, with individualized targets set regarding frequency, type, duration, and intensity. A simple way to start is to ascertain if there is any pregnancy barrier to gentle walking, especially after meals, to reduce postprandial glucose rise, which is a key monitoring time point in GDM.

Target blood glucose levels for pregnant women with GDM are listed in Table 9.3.

TABLE 9.3

Target blood glucose levels for pregnant women

Parameter	Blood glucose (mmol/L)
Fasting	<5.3
1-hour postprandial	<7.8
2-hour postprandial	<6.7

If the woman with GDM does not achieve glycemic targets within 1–2 weeks of initiating lifestyle changes, insulin should be started. Strong consideration should be given to using a basal/bolus insulin regimen, as the bolus premeal insulin most effectively addresses the postprandial glucose rise typically seen in GDM. Understanding the role of insulin resistance in the development of GDM, it is often the postprandial glucose rise that is out of target. Basal insulin at bedtime will manage elevated fasting glucose levels if also present.

Self-monitoring of blood glucose (SMBG) records should be reassessed in a timely fashion, as the window of opportunity is small in pregnancy. It is generally recommended that blood glucose control should be reassessed every 1–2 weeks. Usually, small doses of rapid-acting insulin before meals are sufficient to lower blood glucose levels to target. The rapid-acting analogues lispro, aspart, or glulisine may be used in pregnancy. If fasting blood glucose levels remain out of target, the addition of small doses of bedtime basal insulin should be considered. Basal insulin use often starts with NPH insulin, as it is less expensive and will be used for a limited time over the course of the pregnancy. The long-acting insulin analogues detemir and glargine can also be used. There is no recommendation for degludec insulin at this time but it may be recommended in the future.

A1C is usually checked at the time of diagnosis but is not followed as closely as SMBG records. A change in A1C will be seen too late because of the 3-month turnover for red blood cells.

As pregnant women with GDM are considered to have a somewhat higher-risk pregnancy, increased clinical monitoring by the diabetes and obstetric healthcare teams, as well as fetal assessment, occurs. Delivery is generally planned in advance of the estimated due date, dependent on ongoing blood glucose control.

Postpartum follow-up
Upon delivery, insulin and SMBG may be discontinued. Post partum (between 6 weeks and 6 months), the 75-g 2 hour OGTT should be performed to assess for possible development of prediabetes or T2 diabetes.

Case study
Karen

Karen is a 36-year-old woman who is pregnant with her third child; she is currently at 26 weeks' gestation. She undergoes the standard 1 hour 50-g glucose screen and her blood glucose result is 8.3 mmol/L. As this is considered a positive screen, Karen undergoes a 75-g 2 hour OGTT in a timely fashion. The results are

- Fasting blood glucose, 5.8 mmol/L;
- 1-hour blood glucose, 11.2 mmol/L;
- 2-hour blood glucose, 8.8 mmol/L.

The fasting and 1-hour levels are above the threshold, so a diagnosis of GDM is made.

Karen has at least one recognized risk factor for GDM: her age. She may also have other risk factors, including a family history of T2 diabetes, a history of GDM, and overweight in prepregnancy, which should be ascertained.

Karen wants to understand how this will affect her pregnancy. Karen should be informed that GDM is caused by insulin resistance in later pregnancy secondary to the placental hormones, precipitated by any pre-existing risk factors. GDM can often be modified by changes in nutritional intake and incorporation of moderate physical activity into daily routines.

Karen's GDM changes the status of her pregnancy into a higher risk category. She will benefit from some straightforward nutritional education. She will learn to identify the carbohydrate component of her diet and how to distribute carbohydrate intake evenly throughout the day (ingestion of a large amount of carbohydrate at any single time can result in postprandial hyperglycemia). Moderate physical activity, such as walking after meals, can also reduce postprandial glucose levels.

After 2 weeks, Karen's SMBG records are reviewed. Her 2-hour post-supper glucose levels are above the target of 6.7 mmol/L 85% of the time. Accordingly, her usual supper diet was reviewed for any outstanding sources of carbohydrate. Nothing was identified so she was started on a small dose of rapid-acting insulin at suppertime only. She was instructed to start with 2 units of rapid-acting insulin before supper and to titrate the dose by 1–2 units daily until her 2-hour post-supper glucose levels come into target. At 32 weeks' gestation, Karen's SMBG records indicated that her 2-hour postbreakfast levels were above target the majority of the time; thus 2 units of rapid-acting insulin were added for breakfast in addition to her supper dose, with the same instruction to titrate the dose. Within 2 weeks, Karen was taking 4 units at breakfast and 5 units at supper, which was sufficient to maintain all her blood glucose levels in target for the balance of her pregnancy.

Karen continued her insulin regimen throughout the remainder of her pregnancy and was instructed to discontinue it post partum, as the placental source of insulin resistance was gone. However, Karen still carries a long-term risk of developing T2 diabetes so she was instructed to undergo a 75-g 2 hour OGTT within 6 months' post partum. She was also counseled about healthy eating and physical activity in order to reduce any future risk of GDM or T2 diabetes. In the event that she has a future pregnancy, she should be screened earlier than 26 weeks. Her primary care provider should also screen Karen annually with an A1C looking for prediabetes or T2 diabetes.

Pre-existing diabetes in pregnancy: type 1 or type 2 diabetes

Preconception planning is key in women with pre-existing type 1 (T1) or T2 diabetes. Such planning will optimize glycemic control and assess for the presence of any maternal long-term complications of diabetes.

An elevated A1C can be associated with an increased risk of the development of congenital anomalies. Also, of concern, pregnancy may exacerbate already present long-term complications of retinopathy and nephropathy.

Women with pre-existing diabetes should optimize glycemic control to attain A1C ≤7.0% in order to decrease the risks of congenital malformation, first-trimester spontaneous abortion, preeclampsia, and progression of retinopathy and/or nephropathy. Women with T2 diabetes using antihyperglycemic agents (AHAs) should be transitioned to basal/bolus insulin. Currently, large-scale multicenter clinical studies are being analyzed to assess the addition of metformin to insulin regimens in pre-existing T2 diabetes. At this time, the use of AHAs as first-line therapy in pre-existing T2 diabetes and pregnancy is not recommended.

Preconception planning checklist

- Achieve and maintain target A1C
- Perform retinal assessment
- Determine the presence of microalbuminuria/nephropathy
- Control blood pressure utilizing pregnancy-approved medications
- Discontinue any medications not approved in pregnancy, including angiotensin-converting enzyme inhibitors, angiotensin II receptor blockers, and statins
- Start folic acid at 1 mg daily
- Start enteric-coated ASA between 12 and 16 weeks' gestation to decrease the risk of preeclampsia

Management of pre-existing diabetes in pregnancy

Target blood glucose levels in women with pre-existing diabetes are no different than those in women with GDM (Table 9.4).

First trimester

Insulin sensitivity usually increases; therefore insulin requirements may actually need to be decreased to prevent hypoglycemia.

TABLE 9.4

Target blood glucose levels for pregnant women with pre-existing diabetes

Parameter	Blood glucose (mmol/L)
Fasting	<5.3
1-hour postprandial	<7.8
2-hour postprandial	<6.7

Second and third trimesters

As with all pregnancies, insulin resistance develops, secondary to insulin resistance caused by placental hormones, and insulin requirements can generally be expected to rise. This is similar to the development of GDM in the later second trimester.

All rapid-acting insulin analogues (lispro, aspart, and glulisine) are approved for use during pregnancy in women with pre-existing diabetes. Most basal insulins (e.g., NPH, glargine, and detemir) are approved in pregnancy; however, insulin degludec is not currently approved for this indication but it may be recommended in the future.

As pregnant women with pre-existing diabetes are considered higher risk, increased monitoring is essential; this should include clinical monitoring by the diabetes and obstetric healthcare teams, as well as regular formal ultrasound fetal assessment. Delivery will be planned in advance of the estimated due date, dependent on this monitoring.

Postpartum management

The insulin resistance that occurs during the latter half of pregnancy diminishes immediately after delivery. Therefore it is important to note the prepregnancy insulin dosages and have these women decrease their postpartum dosages to prevent hypoglycemia. Women with T2 diabetes who prefer to restart their AHAs may do so at this time. Breastfeeding is considered safe when using the common AHAs metformin and gliclazide. Currently, there are no recommendations for use of any of the newer AHAs when breastfeeding.

Case study
Lauren

Lauren is a 28-year-old woman who was diagnosed with T1 diabetes 10 years ago. She uses a basal/bolus insulin regimen of glargine and lispro. She comes to your office for a routine assessment. At 7.5%, her A1C is slightly above optimal. She tells you that she and her husband are considering pregnancy and she wonders what she needs to do.

Because preconception planning is very important in helping reduce risks in a pregnancy complicated by diabetes, it is helpful to address this issue with women long before they are considering pregnancy. Elevated A1C at the time of conception increases the risk of congenital anomalies, so one of the first tasks is to work with Lauren to determine when her blood glucose levels are above target and how she can improve them. Ideally, Lauren should wait until her A1C is optimal before trying to conceive.

As pregnancy can affect any underlying diabetic retinopathy, Lauren should have a retinal assessment performed if it has been more than 1–2 years since her last one. If there was previous evidence of diabetic retinopathy, a complete assessment by a retinal specialist at this time would be prudent. Also, she should have a renal screen to determine the presence of diabetic nephropathy; this screen should include a urine albumin-to-creatinine ratio, serum creatinine level, and estimated glomerular filtration rate. Blood pressure levels should also be assessed. Lastly, you will inform Lauren that she should start folic acid supplementation before conception at a dose of 1 mg daily.

Lauren wants to know what to expect throughout the course of her pregnancy. It should be explained that she may be at risk of hypoglycemia during the first trimester because of increased insulin sensitivity; thus she may need to decrease her insulin dosages during this time. Later, toward the end of the second trimester and onward, insulin resistance arising from placental hormones will occur and she can expect to increase her insulin requirements significantly.

Target glucose levels are tighter in pregnancy (Table 9.4) than those in the normal diabetes population. Thus Lauren will be asked to perform SMBG more frequently than she may be accustomed to doing.

With pre-existing diabetes, the pregnancy is considered higher risk so Lauren will need referrals to an endocrinologist, if she doesn't already have one, and an obstetrician for prenatal care and delivery. Also, she should undergo regular fetal assessment through the second and third trimesters.

With pre-existing diabetes, Lauren can expect to deliver before her due date, usually sometime after 36 weeks' gestation, depending on the clinical monitoring results.

As soon as Lauren delivers her baby, her insulin requirements will return to her prepregnancy levels (or even lower) for a short time after the placental source of insulin resistance has gone. Thus Lauren will need to monitor her blood glucose levels carefully and readjust her insulin dosage as necessary. It helps if Lauren keeps a record of her prepregnancy insulin dosages as a guide. Her insulin dosages will change so often throughout the pregnancy that she may not actually remember her original dosages.

DIABETES CARE IN THE HOSPITAL

Abstract

Diabetes care in various hospital settings, e.g., the emergency room and internal medicine and surgical wards, can be difficult to maintain. Many variables need to be considered, including the stress of an acute illness, which can result in hyperglycemia; disrupted meal, activity, and sleep patterns; intermittent fasting for various procedures; and the complications of hospitalization, particularly infection. Often diabetes management is forgotten in the event of an acute illness, which can lead to diabetes becoming a major problem with the development of hypo- or hyperglycemia. This chapter describes a practical approach to diabetes in various hospital settings, with checklists to help minimize the effect of diabetes in hospital. Methods to dose subcutaneous insulin and insulin infusions are discussed. Pitfalls to a stable diabetes hospital care are identified, and strategies to avoid them are also detailed.

Keywords: Discharge planning; In-hospital blood glucose targets; Insulin correction; Insulin infusion.

Practical Diabetes Care for Healthcare Professionals
ISBN 978-0-12-820082-7
https://doi.org/10.1016/B978-0-12-820082-7.00010-5

Introduction

In my many years of experience consulting about diabetes in hospital, I have witnessed diabetes management that has ranged from "the good, to the bad, to the ugly." Unfortunately, it is the patients with diabetes who suffer the most, as they are buffeted by swinging blood glucose levels while trying to recover from illness or surgery.

I believe that hospital management of diabetes neither has to result in such poor experiences for patients nor has to be complicated for medical staff to manage. There is a logical approach to diabetes hospital management that will help medical staff improve the hospital experience for patients with diabetes.

With this in mind, this chapter is intended for use by the following healthcare professionals working on hospital wards:

- Attending physicians
- Medical trainees
- Physician assistants
- Clinical assistants
- Nurse practitioners
- Nurses
- Dietitians
- Allied healthcare professionals

As the prevalence of diabetes is increasing throughout the world, it stands to reason that more patients who are admitted to hospital have diabetes. If it is considered by either the patient or the medical staff to be a minor medical problem and placed at the bottom of a long list of medical issues, then be warned! Diabetes can easily rise to the top of that list, causing complications that may significantly worsen and prolong the patient's hospital stay. Poorly controlled diabetes in one hospital admission can, unfortunately, be the cause of subsequent and perhaps more complicated admissions. With consistent attention to the basic principles of diabetes management and some exercise of logic and common sense, diabetes-related complications, particularly iatrogenic complications, can be reduced significantly.

It is important to understand that the best advocate for optimal diabetes management is the patient! The person with diabetes best understands their diabetes. Many patients have been well educated about the concept of diabetes self-management and have been directing their own diabetes management for years. Imagine such an individual entering hospital and losing that control. It is bad enough to lose control over their health—whether they are now ill with pneumonia, myocardial infarction, or a broken leg—now they have lost control of their diabetes management, their medication or insulin regimen, their eating habits, and their exercise routine. Worse yet, they feel that they are at the mercy of someone they would rightfully consider far less knowledgeable in managing their diabetes in hospital.

All people admitted to hospital are stressed. By its broadest definition, stress encompasses factors such as the anxiety and fear of illness, disruptive sleep and wake cycles, pain, shortness of breath, and the body's inflammatory response to all these factors. Part of the body's response to stress includes the increase of the counterregulatory hormones catecholamine, cortisol, growth hormone, and glucagon. These hormones all share the property of increasing blood glucose levels. Add to that stress-induced hyperglycemia, bed rest with inactivity, glucose-containing intravenous (IV) solutions, the use of tube feeds (TF) or total parenteral nutrition (TPN), or the use of drugs known to increase blood glucose levels (e.g., corticosteroids), and the makings of a hyperglycemia "perfect storm" are present.

Further complicating diabetes management in hospital is the fact that the most common acute adverse effect in people with diabetes who are hospitalized is hypoglycemia, not hyperglycemia. Consider the reasons for this. First, most patients have a decreased appetite. By nature, the hospital diet is strict in calories but often wanting in taste, due to the necessary requirements for salt and fat restrictions. Furthermore, an institutional kitchen is simply not equipped to produce restaurant-quality meals. Lastly, many patients simply do not have an appetite while they are ill.

Added to this setting is the innate desire of healthcare professionals to "fix" what appears to be "broken": infection, chest pain, coronary artery disease, broken leg, and, of course, blood glucose levels. It has been well recognized that guideline-recommended optimal diabetes control is the target thought to be attained in hospital, which means blood glucose levels between 4.0 and 7.0 mmol/L before meals. If a patient's blood glucose level is high, the overwhelming desire on the part of the medical staff is to lower it. Insulin is dispensed quite freely, usually in aliquots of 5 units, which somehow conveys the false message of appropriate diabetes management. At the very least, it keeps the number of calls from the ward staff to a minimum but, in reality, intermittent dosages of insulin result in worsening blood glucose control, not better.

Finally, there is the scenario that is most inappropriate for someone with diabetes, i.e., the attempt to establish "good" glucose control in hospital. There are probably still instances where a patient is admitted to achieve diabetes control. For all these reasons stated above, it is virtually impossible to establish good diabetes control in hospital. To attempt to do so is usually an exercise in futility for patient and staff alike.

So why bother attempting to maintain appropriate blood glucose control in hospital? There is more than sufficient evidence to show the harm that hyperglycemia can cause in a hospitalized patient. The presence of hyperglycemia in a septic patient will both prolong and decrease healing and may actually be the root cause of septic complications in both surgical and nonsurgical patients. However, the ad hoc use of insulin to control hyperglycemia without a logical approach will inevitably result in hypo-glycemia, the most common complication affecting people with diabetes in hospital. Often, the result is blood glucose levels that swing between high and low. Unfortunately, as the blood glucose swings, so does the patient. The ill effects and symptoms of highs and lows, and all the swinging in between, have now been added to their illness.

The first principle in managing diabetes in hospital is to determine appropriate target blood glucose levels, i.e., blood glucose levels that will prevent the acute complications of either hypo- or hyperglycemia. For most patients, this translates to a range of 5.0/6.0—10.0/12.0 mmol/L. This range will maintain good polymorphonuclear (white blood) cell function against infection, while avoiding acute complications. For more critically ill patients, this target can be adjusted to 6.0/8.0—10.0 mmol/L, depending on the availability of nursing staff to monitor blood glucose levels as needed.

The advent of rapid-acting insulins, which start working within 15 minutes, peak at 90—120 minutes, and are virtually cleared from the body after 2—3 hours, have heralded a new era of much easier blood glucose control. Rapid-acting insulins reduce the risk of hypoglycemia, as they have a shorter duration of action than regular insulin and, accordingly, are usually given with meals.

Just say no to the sliding scale

Rapid-acting insulins are also effective for use as a corrective measure, aka correction factor (CF), to maintain optimal blood glucose targets for patients in hospital. This approach replaces the commonly used (and, in my opinion, misused) insulin sliding scale. Sliding scales represent a reactive, rather than a proactive, approach to blood glucose control. They deliver variable amounts of insulin at variable times, generally resulting in those swinging blood glucose levels. Instead, the use of a rapid-acting insulin CF at mealtimes alongside an established diabetes medication regimen will result in much smoother blood glucose control. The application of this principle will be explained for each hospital setting.

Acute illness and antihyperglycemic agents

The use of a number of antihyperglycemic agents (AHAs) should be stopped temporarily in the presence of any acute intercurrent illness, as they can either worsen the illness or cause other complications themselves.

- Sodium glucose co-transporter 2 (SGLT2) inhibitors
  - They can lead to dehydration, which can in turn lead to postural dizziness or syncope.
  - Euglycemic diabetic ketoacidosis (DKA) is a rare adverse complication that occurs at blood glucose levels lower than those in other presentations of DKA; euglycemic DKA is often precipitated by an intercurrent illness.
- Metformin
  - If an intercurrent illness leads to dehydration and a prerenal state, clearance of metformin decreases.
  - In the presence of decreased renal function or very low cardiac ejection fraction (severe congestive heart failure), clearance of metformin further decreases and may also lead to the rare complication of lactic acidosis.
  - It is recommended that for estimated glomerular filtration rate (eGFR) 30–60 mL/min/1.73 m^2, dosage should be limited to 500 mg bid; for eGFR <30 mL/min/1.73 m^2, metformin administration should be stopped.
- Sulfonylureas
  - They can precipitate hypoglycemia.

Other medications often used in diabetes, including angiotensin-converting enzyme inhibitors, angiotensin II receptor blockers, diuretics, and direct renin inhibitors, may also worsen the intercurrent illness. The mnemonic SADMANS (Fig. 10.1) is commonly used to identify those medication categories that should be temporarily stopped in the presence of acute illness.

FIGURE 10.1

SADMANS

S	Sulfonylureas
A	ACE inhibitors
D	Diuretics, direct renin inhibitors
M	Metformin
A	ARB
N	Nonsteroidal anti-inflammatory agents
S	SGLT2 inhibitors

Source: Reproduced with permission from Diabetes Canada 2018 Clinical Practice Guidelines for the Prevention and Management of Diabetes in Canada.
ACE, angiotensin-converting enzyme; ARB, angiotensin II receptor blocker; SGLT2, sodium glucose co-transporter 2.

Table 10.1 offers a review of available AHAs and insulin. It is important to recognize their mechanisms of action and how they could impact patients in hospital.

Fig. 10.2 identifies dosage adjustment for eGFR for all classes of diabetes medication, including insulin.

Table 10.2 identifies the various insulin types available, and Fig. 10.3 depicts rapid- and long-acting insulin action profiles. It is important to realize that there is a significant difference between rapid- and short-acting insulin with respect to time to onset and duration of action.

The following is a set of assumptions or understandings regarding hospital management of patients with diabetes:

- Acute illness generally results in hyperglycemia.
- More stable conditions may result in hypoglycemia when the preadmission diabetes medications and dosages are continued in the presence of the calorie- and/or carbohydrate (CHO)-controlled hospital diabetes diet.
- It is important to individualize safe target blood glucose ranges for hospitalized patients.
- Hospital is not the setting to establish optimal blood glucose control.
- Above all else, remember that hypoglycemia causes more harm in hospital than hyperglycemia.

TABLE 10.1

Antihyperglycemic agents

Agent	Mechanism of action	Dosage	Action time	Benefits	Disadvantages
Biguanide (insulin sensitizer)					
Metformin (Glucophage)	• Insulin sensitizer • Reduces hepatic glucose output	• Start 250–500 mg bid ac meals • Start with low dose and increase slowly • Maximum dose 2550 mg/day in divided doses	8 hours	• Does not promote weight gain • Rarely causes hypoglycemia • Can be used in combination with daytime insulin	• GI: nausea, bloating, diarrhea • Slow increase in dose decreases these side effects: "start low, go slow" • Contraindicated in renal impairment (eGFR <30 mL/min/1.73 m^2), hepatic impairment, or CHF • Maximum dose of 500 mg bid with eGFR 30–60 mL/min/1.73 m^2
Sulfonylureas (insulin secretagogues)					
Glyburide (Diabeta, Glibenclamide)	• Stimulates pancreatic secretion of insulin	• Start at 2.5–5 mg od or bid ac meals • Maximum dose, 10 mg bid	16–24 hours	• Sulfonylureas are often the most potent AHA class	• May cause weight gain • May cause hypoglycemia

Continued

TABLE 10.1

Antihyperglycemic agents—cont'd

Agent	Mechanism of action	Dosage	Action time	Benefits	Disadvantages
Gliclazide (Diamicron)	• Stimulates pancreatic secretion of insulin	• Start at 80 mg od • Maximum dose, 160 mg bid	8–16 hours	• Causes less hypoglycemia than glyburide	• May cause weight gain
Gliclazide MR (Diamicron MR)	• Stimulates pancreatic secretion of insulin	• Start at 30 mg od • Maximum dose, 120 mg od	24 hours	• Causes less hypoglycemia than glyburide	• May cause weight gain
Glimepiride (Amaryl)	• Stimulates pancreatic secretion of insulin	• Start at 1–2 mg od • Dosage range: 1–8 mg od	24 hours	• May be used in combination with daytime insulin • May cause less hypoglycemia than glyburide	• May cause weight gain
α-Glucosidase inhibitor					
Acarbose (Prandase, Glucobay)	• Inhibits glucosidase enzymes in CHO digestion • Decreases postprandial glucose rise	• Start at 25 mg with first bite of food • Titrate weekly to usual dose of 50–100 mg/meal	Best effect seen postprandially	• No hypoglycemia if used alone	• GI: bloating, flatus • Start with low dose and increase slowly to decrease GI side effects • Beano counteracts glucose effects • When treating hypoglycemia use dextrose tablets, milk, or honey

Meglitinide (insulin secretagogue)

Repaglinide (GlucoNorm)	• Stimulates pancreatic insulin secretion • Different mechanisms of action than sulfonylureas	• Start at 0.5 mg 0–30 minutes before each meal • Or titrate according to CHO intake (1 mg/15 g CHO) • Available in 0.5, 1, and 2 mg dosages	Short-acting; stimulates insulin secretion in response to glucose rise at mealtime	• Controls postprandial glucose rise • Provides flexibility to fit varied mealtimes	• May cause hypoglycemia

Thiazolidinediones (insulin sensitizers)

Rosiglitazone (Avandia)	• Insulin sensitizer • Insulin action improved in liver, muscle, and adipose tissue	• 2–8 mg daily as a bid dosage	Effect seen after 6 weeks	• May increase TG and decrease HDL levels	• May cause weight gain, peripheral edema, macular edema, or CHF • Rare occurrence of osteoporosis in women • Contraindicated in CHF, hepatic impairment (monitor liver function test results regularly) • Should not be used in combination with daytime insulin • Rosiglitazone, alone or in combination, is prescribed with both physician and patient waivers

Continued

TABLE 10.1

Antihyperglycemic agents—cont'd

Agent	Mechanism of action	Dosage	Action time	Benefits	Disadvantages
Rosiglitazone/metformin (Avandamet)	• As per rosiglitazone and metformin	• Rosiglitazone: 1–4 mg • Metformin: 500–1000 mg	4–6 weeks	• As per rosiglitazone and metformin	• As per rosiglitazone and metformin
Rosiglitazone/glimepiride (Avandaryl)	• As per rosiglitazone and glimepiride	• Rosiglitazone: 1–4 mg • Glimepiride: 1, 2, or 4 mg	4–6 weeks	• As per rosiglitazone and glimepiride	• As per rosiglitazone and glimepiride
Pioglitazone (Actos)	• Insulin sensitizer • Insulin action improved in liver, muscle, and adipose tissue	• 15–45 mg daily	4–6 weeks	• As per rosiglitazone	• As per rosiglitazone • May be associated with a risk of bladder cancer • Does not require waiver for prescription

Drug	Mechanism	Dosage	Titration	Benefits	Considerations
Pioglitazone/ metformin (Actoplus Met)	• As per pioglitazone and metformin	• Pioglitazone: 15 mg • Metformin: 500 and 850 mg	4–6 weeks	• As per pioglitazone and metformin	• As per pioglitazone and metformin
Pioglitazone/ glimepiride (Duetact)	• As per metformin and glimepiride	• Pioglitazone: 30 mg • Glimepiride: 2 and 4 mg	4–6 weeks	• As per pioglitazone and glimepiride	• As per pioglitazone and glimepiride
Incretins (augment insulin action)					
Sitagliptin (Januvia)	• Augments endogenous insulin • Blocks glucagon action in liver • Sensitizer and secretagogue effects	• 100 mg daily (50 mg daily with renal impairment)	4–6 weeks	• Weight neutral • Low risk for hypoglycemia	• Rare risk of pancreatitis • Contraindicated in those with a history of medullary thyroid cancer/multiple endocrine neoplasia • Requires dosage reduction in the presence of CKD

Continued

TABLE 10.1

Antihyperglycemic agents—cont'd

Agent	Mechanism of action	Dosage	Action time	Benefits	Disadvantages
Sitagliptin/metformin (Janumet)	• As per sitagliptin and metformin	• Sitagliptin: 50 mg • Metformin: 500–1000 mg	As per sitagliptin and metformin	• As per sitagliptin and metformin	• As per sitagliptin and metformin
Saxagliptin (Onglyza)	• Augments endogenous insulin • Blocks glucagon action in liver • Sensitizer and secretagogue effects	• 5 mg daily	4–6 weeks	• Weight neutral	• Rare risk of pancreatitis • Contraindicated in those with a history of medullary thyroid cancer/multiple endocrine neoplasia • Requires dosage reduction in the presence of CKD
Saxagliptin/metformin (Kombiglyze)	• As per saxagliptin and metformin	• Saxagliptin: 2.5, 5 mg • Metformin: 500 and 1000 mg	4–6 weeks	• As per saxagliptin and metformin	• As per saxagliptin and metformin

Linagliptin (Trajenta)	• Augments endogenous insulin • Blocks glucagon action in liver • Sensitizer and secretagogue effects	• 5 mg daily	4–6 weeks	• Does not require dosage adjustment in the presence of CKD	• Rare risk of pancreatitis • Contraindicated in those with a history of medullary thyroid cancer/multiple endocrine neoplasia • No dosage reduction until an eGFR of 15 mL/min/1.73 m^2
Linagliptin/metformin (Jentadueto)	• Augments endogenous insulin • Blocks glucagon action in liver • Sensitizer and secretagogue effects	• Linagliptin: 2.5 mg • Metformin: 500, 850, and 1000 mg	4–6 weeks	• Does not require dosage adjustment in the presence of CKD	• As per linagliptin and metformin

Continued

TABLE 10.1

Antihyperglycemic agents—cont'd

Agent	Mechanism of action	Dosage	Action time	Benefits	Disadvantages
GLP-1 receptor agonists (augment endogenous insulin)					
Liraglutide (Victoza)	• Augments endogenous insulin • Blocks glucagon action in liver • Sensitizer and secretagogue effects	0.6–1.8 sc mg daily	4–6 weeks	• Weight neutral • May lead to weight loss • Indications for CVD and renal benefits	• May cause nausea • Rare risk of pancreatitis • Contraindicated in those with a history of medullary thyroid cancer/multiple endocrine neoplasia • Not advised when eGFR <15 mL/min/1.73 m^2
Lixisenatide daily (Adlyxine)	• Augments endogenous insulin • Blocks glucagon action in liver • Sensitizer and secretagogue effects	10 µg sc od for 14 days then titrate to maintenance dose of 20 µg od	4–6 weeks	• Weight neutral • May lead to weight loss	• May cause nausea • Rare risk of pancreatitis • Contraindicated in those with a history of medullary thyroid cancer/multiple endocrine neoplasia • Contraindicated when eGFR <30 mL/min/1.73 m^2

Exenatide (extended release) (Bydureon)	• Augments endogenous insulin • Blocks glucagon action in liver • Sensitizer and secretagogue effects	2 mg sc weekly	4–6 weeks	• Weight neutral • May lead to weight loss	• May cause nausea • Rare risk of pancreatitis • Contraindicated in those with a history of medullary thyroid cancer/multiple endocrine neoplasia • Caution when eGFR <50 mL/min/ 1.73 m² and stop if eGFR <30 mL/min/ 1.73 m²
Dulaglutide weekly (Trulicity)	• Augments endogenous insulin • Blocks glucagon action in liver • Sensitizer and secretagogue effects	0.75 mg weekly, which can be titrated to 1.5 mg weekly after 1–2 weeks	4–6 weeks	• Weight neutral • May lead to weight loss • Indications for CVD and renal benefits	• May cause nausea • Rare risk of pancreatitis • Contraindicated in those with a history of medullary thyroid cancer/multiple endocrine neoplasia • Caution when eGFR <15 mL/min/ 1.73 m²

Continued

TABLE 10.1

Antihyperglycemic agents—cont'd

Agent	Mechanism of action	Dosage	Action time	Benefits	Disadvantages
Semaglutide weekly (Ozempic)	• Augments endogenous insulin • Blocks glucagon action in liver • Sensitizer and secretagogue effects	• 0.25 mg sc weekly • After 4 weeks the dose should be increased to 0.5 mg sc weekly • Additional titration may be increased to 1 mg once weekly	4–6 weeks	• Weight neutral • May lead to weight loss • Shown to have CVD and renal benefits	• May cause nausea • Rare risk of pancreatitis • Contraindicated in those with a history of medullary thyroid cancer/multiple endocrine neoplasia • Caution when eGFR <15 mL/min/1.73 m^2
Semaglutide daily (Rybelsus)	• Augments endogenous insulin • Blocks glucagon action in liver • Sensitizer and secretagogue effects	• 3 mg po daily • After 30 days may increase to 7 mg po daily • Additional titration to 14 mg daily may be increased after another 30 days	4–6 weeks	• Oral medication • Weight neutral • May lead to weight loss • May also have CVD and renal benefits	• May cause nausea • Rare risk of pancreatitis • Contraindicated in those with past history of medullary thyroid cancer/multiple endocrine neoplasia • Caution when eGFR <15 mL/min/1.73 m^2

SGLT2 inhibitors

Canagliflozin (Invokana)	• Inhibits renal reabsorption of glucose	• 100–300 mg daily	4–6 weeks	• May cause modest weight loss • Indications for CVD and renal benefits • Now indicated to continue in patients with eGFR ≥15 mL/min/1.73 m^2	• Glycosuria may increase risk of GU mycotic infections • Rare risk of perineal infections • Risk of dehydration, particularly in elderly and/or in those who use diuretics • Rare risk of euglycemic DKA, should be discontinued with intercurrent illness • Earlier study indicating increased risk of toe amputation but not confirmed in later study • Not advised when eGFR <15 mL/min/1.73 m^2
Canagliflozin/ Metformin (Invokamet)	• As per canagliflozin and metformin	• Canagliflozin: 50 and 150 mg • Metformin: 500 and 1000 mg	4–6 weeks	• As per canagliflozin and metformin	• As per canagliflozin and metformin
Dapagliflozin (Forxiga)	• Inhibits renal reabsorption of glucose	• 5–10 mg daily	6 weeks	• May cause modest weight loss • Shown to have benefits in congestive heart failure	• Glycosuria may increase risk of GU mycotic infections • Rare risk of perineal infections • Risk of dehydration, particularly in elderly and/or in those who use diuretics

Continued

TABLE 10.1

Antihyperglycemic agents—cont'd

Agent	Mechanism of action	Dosage	Action time	Benefits	Disadvantages
					• Rare risk of euglycemic DKA, should be discontinued with intercurrent illness • Caution with decreased renal function
Dapagliflozin/ metformin (Xigduo)	• As per dapagliflozin and metformin	• Dapagliflozin: 5 and 10 mg • Metformin: 500 and 1000 mg	4–6 weeks	• As per dapagliflozin and metformin	• As per dapagliflozin and metformin
Empagliflozin (Jardiance)	• Inhibits renal reabsorption of glucose	• 10–25 mg daily	4–6 weeks	• May cause modest weight loss • Indications for CVD and renal benefit	• Glycosuria may increase risk of GU mycotic infections • Rare risk of perineal infections • Risk of dehydration, particularly in elderly and/or in those who use diuretics • Rare risk of euglycemic DKA, should be discontinued with intercurrent illness • Caution with decreased renal function

Drug	Mechanism	Dose	Titration	Benefits	Risks/Considerations
Empagliflozin/metformin (Synjardy)	• As per empagliflozin and metformin	• Empagliflozin: 5 and 12.5 mg • Metformin: 500 and 1000 mg	4–6 weeks	• As per empagliflozin and metformin	• As per empagliflozin and metformin
Empagliflozin/metformin extended release (Synjardy XR)	• As per empagliflozin and metformin	• Empagliflozin: 5, 10, and 12.5 mg • Metformin: 1000 mg	4–6 weeks	• As per empagliflozin and metformin	• As per empagliflozin and metformin
Ertugliflozin (Steglatro)	• Inhibits renal reabsorption of glucose	• 5–15 mg daily	4–6 weeks	• May cause modest weight loss • No evidence yet for CVD or renal benefits	• Glycosuria may increase risk of GU mycotic infections • Rare risk of perineal infections • Risk of dehydration, particularly in elderly and/or in those who use diuretics • Rare risk of euglycemic DKA, should be discontinued with intercurrent illness • Contraindicated when eGFR <45 mL/min/1.73 m^2

Continued

TABLE 10.1

Antihyperglycemic agents—cont'd

Agent	Mechanism of action	Dosage	Action time	Benefits	Disadvantages
Sotagliflozin (Zynquista in the European Union; not yet approved in North America)	• As per ertugliflozin	• 200–400 mg OD	• 4–6 weeks	• Recent studies have indicated possible benefit for CVD and hospitalization for congestive heart failure	• Glycosuria may increase risk of GU mycotic infections • Rare risk of perineal infections • Risk of dehydration, particularly in elderly and/or in those who use diuretics • Rare risk of euglycemic DKA, should be discontinued with intercurrent illness • Caution with decreased renal function
Dopamine agonist (novel use for diabetes)					
Bromocriptine-QR (Cycloset)		• 0.8 mg daily, titrated weekly to 1.6–4.8 mg			• Nausea • Postural dizziness
Weight loss agent					
Orlistat (Xenical)	• Inhibits lipase	• 100 mg with each meal			• Adverse GI effects

Insulin/AHA combinations

Insulin glargine/ lixisenatide (Soliqua)	Lixisenatide actions: • Augments endogenous insulin • Blocks glucagon action in liver • Therefore both sensitizer and secretagogue effects Glargine actions: • Refer to insulin section	• Therapy with basal insulin should be discontinued prior to initiation of Soliqua • In patients inadequately controlled on <30 units of basal insulin, the recommended starting dosage of Soliqua is 15 units (15 units glargine/ 5 µg lixisenatide) given sc once daily • Titration according to FPG by 2–4 units insulin/week • Titration of insulin automatically changes lixisenatide dose	1–2 weeks	• As per lixisenatide and glargine	• As per lixisenatide and glargine

Continued

TABLE 10.1

Antihyperglycemic agents—cont'd

Agent	Mechanism of action	Dosage	Action time	Benefits	Disadvantages
Insulin degludec/ liraglutide (Xultophy)	Liraglutide actions: • Augments endogenous insulin • Blocks glucagon action in liver • Therefore both sensitizer and secretagogue effects Degludec actions: • Refer to insulin section	• Basal insulin therapy should be discontinued prior to initiation of Xultophy • In patients inadequately controlled on <50 units of basal insulin or liraglutide (≤1.8 g daily) the recommended starting dosage is as follows: • New start: 10 units of insulin degludec and 0.36 mg liraglutide • Converting from basal insulin or liraglutide: 16 units of insulin degludec and 0.58 mg liraglutide	1–2 weeks	• As per liraglutide and degludec	• As per liraglutide and degludec

- Dose may be titrated twice/weekly by 1–2 units of insulin as the liraglutide will automatically change according to FPG to a maximum of 50/1.8 mg

ac, before meals; AHA, antihyperglycemic agent; bid, twice daily; CHF, congestive heart failure; CHO, carbohydrate; CKD, chronic kidney disease; CVD, cardiovascular disease; DKA, diabetic ketoacidosis; eGFR, estimated glomerular filtration rate; FPG, fasting plasma glucose; GI, gastrointestinal; GLP-1, glucagon-like peptide 1; GU, genitourinary; HDL, high-density lipoprotein; od, once daily; sc, subcutaneously; SGLT2, sodium glucose co-transporter 2; TG, triglyceride; tid, three times daily.

FIGURE 10.2

Antihyperglycemic agents and dose adjustment for renal function

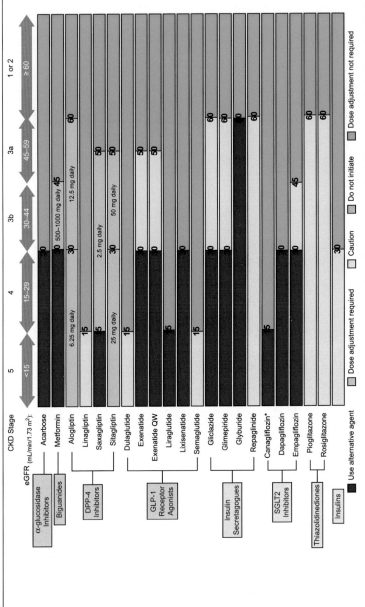

Source: *Reproduced with permission from Diabetes Canada 2018 Clinical Practice Guidelines for the Prevention and Management of Diabetes in Canada.*
CKD, chronic kidney disease; CVD, cardiovascular disease; DPP-4, dipeptidyl peptidase-4; eGFR, estimated glomerular filtration rate; GLP-1, glucagon-like peptide 1; SGLT2, sodium glucose co-transporter 2.

TABLE 10.2

Insulin types

Type	Trade name	Onset	Peak	Duration
Rapid-acting (analogue)				
Aspart, ultrarapid-acting	Fiasp	4—5 minutes	1.0—1.5 hours	2—4 hours
Lispro (U-100 or U-200)	Humalog	10—15 minutes		
Aspart	NovoRapid	10—15 minutes		
Glulisine	Apidra	10—15 minutes		
Short-acting (human)				
Regular	Humulin R	0.5—1 hours	2—4 hours	6—8 hours
	Novolin ge			
	Toronto			
Intermediate-acting (human)				
NPH	Humulin N	1—3 hours	4—8 hours	12—16 hours
Long-acting (analogue)				
Glargine	Lantus	90 minutes	No peak	24 hours
U-300 glargine	Toujeo			
Detemir	Levemir			
Degludec (U-100 or U-200)	Tresiba			>24 hours

Continued

TABLE 10.2

Insulin types—cont'd

Type	Trade name	Onset	Peak	Duration
Premixed (short- and intermediate-acting, R/NPH) (human)				
30/70 40/60 50/50	Humulin (30/70 only) Novolin ge	0.5 hours	2–12 hours 2–3 hours 1 hour	12–18 hours
Premixed insulin (rapid- and intermediate-acting) (analogue)				
25% rapid-acting/75% intermediate-acting 30% rapid-acting/70% intermediate-acting 50% rapid-acting/50% intermediate-acting	Humalog Mix 25 NovoMix 70/30 Mix 50	15 minutes	90 minutes–4 hours	10–14 hours

NPH, neutral protamine Hagedorn; *R*, regular insulin.

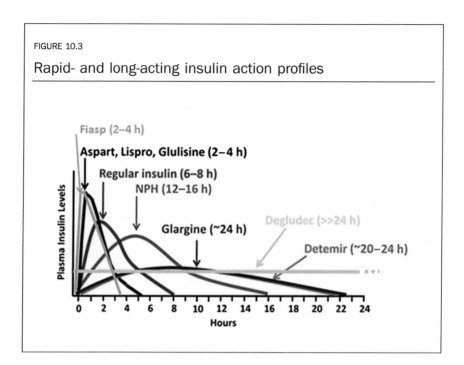

FIGURE 10.3

Rapid- and long-acting insulin action profiles

Fiasp (2–4 h)

Aspart, Lispro, Glulisine (2–4 h)

Regular insulin (6–8 h)

NPH (12–16 h)

Glargine (~24 h)

Degludec (>>24 h)

Detemir (~20–24 h)

Plasma Insulin Levels

0 2 4 6 8 10 12 14 16 18 20 22 24

Hours

Diabetes in the emergency room

Please note that this chapter does not address the management of the acute complications of DKA or hyperglycemic hyperosmolar nonketotic states, which are addressed in the Acute Complications of Diabetes chapter. Rather, it is meant to identify and help avoid the pitfalls that can complicate the situation of people with diabetes who are admitted to the emergency room (ER) for other reasons.

People with diabetes are at greater risk for a variety of acute medical events, including sepsis, cardiovascular disease, acute myocardial infarction, and renal disease. Thus diabetes will be on the problem list of many ER patients. However, in the chaos that typifies the ER, patients' diabetes—or more, importantly, their blood glucose status—may be temporarily neglected as their more emergent issues are dealt with. Diabetes, if left poorly controlled, can complicate almost any medical condition and lead to the development of further medical problems, particularly sepsis.

A quick survey of every patient, asking whether they have diabetes, would be useful. For those with diabetes, a quick further inquiry regarding their medication regimen (oral agents or insulin) and, perhaps more importantly, when they last took their medication does not take much time and can provide important information to prevent further acute diabetes complications.

Here is a sample of a useful quick survey regarding a patient's diabetes status:

- Do you know if you have type 1 (T1) or type 2 (T2) diabetes? (Remember, the use of insulin does not differentiate T1 from T2 diabetes.)
- What medications, pills and/or insulin, do you take for your diabetes?
- What diabetes medications did you take today? At what time did you take them?
- When was your last blood glucose reading? What was the reading?
- Have you been able to eat? When did you last eat?

If people with diabetes are without their diabetes medications, they will become increasingly hyperglycemic and will be open to the risk of metabolic derangements, particularly DKA in those with T1 diabetes. Thus there is a need for increased advocacy for the patient with diabetes in the ER. This may come from the patient, their family, or healthcare staff. It is of benefit to all to listen and pay attention to the patient's diabetes status. Simple maintenance of an appropriate blood glucose range will decrease the risk of a more complicated hospital stay.

A practical approach for blood glucose control in the emergency room

- Set a target blood glucose range that is appropriate for the situation: 6.0—12.0 mmol/L.
- For stable patients who can eat, continue their diabetes medication regimen and use glucose monitoring to maintain the target glucose range.
- Supplement with the use of the following *rapid-acting* insulin CF every 4—6 hours to maintain target blood glucose level: give 1—2 units of *rapid-acting* insulin for every 3.0 mmol/L blood glucose level greater than 12.0 mmol/L.
- Patients must have a source of food/glucose, either oral or IV.

- For patients with significantly acute illness who cannot eat, use the *rapid-acting* insulin CF or consider establishing an insulin infusion:
  - Start with *regular/rapid-acting* insulin at 1 unit/hour with a simultaneous glucose infusion (5% dextrose and water [D5W] at 50–75 cc/hour). The D5W provides not only some CHO substrate for the insulin but also a safety measure to avoid insulin left running unopposed by any glucose.
  - Titrate the insulin ±1 unit/hour to maintain target blood glucose range.

Case study
Evelyn

Evelyn is a 75-year-old woman with longstanding T2 diabetes. She takes gliclazide MR 90 mg od and metformin 850 mg tid. She presents in the evening with sepsis, which may be caused by a urinary tract infection. She is vomiting and not eating. She did not take her diabetes medications today and her blood glucose level is 22.0 mmol/L. She is started on IV fluids, D5W/1/2 NS at 100 cc/hour and IV antibiotics. She is to be reassessed tomorrow.

The concerns here are the risk of continued hyperglycemia complicating her sepsis, her inability to keep food down, and her medication. Do not forget, metformin must be reevaluated in the presence of possible dehydration, causing a rise in serum creatinine levels.

A logical approach would be one of the following:
- *Discontinue all oral diabetes medications,*
- *Perform regular blood glucose monitoring every 2 hours,*
- *Use the rapid-acting insulin CF every 4–6 hours,*

or
- *Start an insulin infusion until Evelyn is able to tolerate oral fluids and medications once again (see Insulin Infusions section).*

Diabetes on the medical ward

Clinical experience has shown that blood glucose levels swing, often quite widely, on the internal medical ward. Unfortunately, these swings are often iatrogenic in nature. Fortunately, however, iatrogenic causes can be fixed through an understanding of the basic reason for blood glucose variability in the hospital ward and the application of a few general principles.

In the acute phase of illness and hospitalization with elevation of stress responses, blood glucose levels tend to rise; in the longer, more stable, hospitalization, blood glucose levels tend to drop in response to the CHO-controlled hospital diet. Usual sleep/wake cycles are disrupted, thereby increasing both stress and blood glucose levels. Inactivity can also increase blood glucose levels. The timing of meals and snacks will vary from the patient's home routine. Often, it is the lack of appreciation for the seemingly small details that can result in major problems. For example, on most wards, supper is served at 6:00 P.M. and may be the last food a patient eats until morning. If they receive insulin, secretagogue AHAs, or long-acting insulin at supper or bedtime, there is now a real risk for nocturnal hypoglycemia. In fact, hypoglycemia is a more serious problem on hospital wards than is hyperglycemia. Yet, it seems that hyperglycemia is chased with variable amounts of insulin around the clock, resulting in those infamous blood glucose swings.

In order to achieve stable diabetes control on the ward consider the key understanding noted earlier: *it is important to determine a safe target blood glucose range for the individual hospitalized patient*. An appropriate target range that will avoid the acute problems of hyper- or hypoglycemia is 5.0/6.0–10.0/12.0 mmol/L. This target range will decrease the risk of hyper-glycemia contributing to a risk of sepsis and avoid the risks of hypoglycemia.

A practical approach to blood glucose control in the medical ward
For stable, less acutely ill patients utilize the patient's usual diabetes regimen with dosage adjustments as required. Some patients will need an increase in their dosage of ∼ 10%–15% to accommodate the initial stress hyperglycemia of hospitalization. Remember, however, that once the situation has stabilized, there will likely be a need to reduce the dosage by at least 15%–20% to account for the CHO-controlled hospital diet.

Use the rapid-acting insulin CF at mealtimes to maintain the target blood glucose range as follows:
- Give 1–2 units for every 3.0 mmol/L >12.0 mmol/L (the upper target range). This CF can be used with any existing diabetes regimen.
- Avoid giving rapid-acting insulin CF at bedtime, as this will increase the risk of hypoglycemia.

Insulin sliding scales and why the author hates them!
Insulin sliding scales deliver variable dosages of insulin at variable times, as determined solely by a blood glucose reading. Overall, it is *reactive* to the

last blood glucose value rather than being *proactive* toward the *next* blood glucose value. No other variables are taken into consideration (e.g., time of day). Thus a dose of insulin may be given at night when the patient will have no food intake until morning. Or, another dose of insulin may be administered on top of a previously ordered dose of oral agent or insulin. So, in effect, insulin and/or oral agents may "stack" on top of each other. Thus sliding scales contain all the ingredients for a perfect storm, resulting in wildly swinging glucose levels.

The rapid-acting insulin CF, given at the usual mealtimes (i.e. insulin administration times), is preferred because it is a proactive, rather than reactive, approach. It builds on an already established diabetes regimen and works to keep the patient's blood glucose level in the designated target range.

Insulin infusions
Acutely ill patients who are unable to eat are best controlled by insulin infusion:

- Start with regular/rapid-acting insulin at 1 unit/hour IV simultaneously running with D5W at 50–75 cc/hour. The D5W provides not only some CHO substrate for the insulin but also a safety measure to avoid insulin left running unopposed by any glucose. Titrate the insulin infusion ±1 unit/hour at a time until the target blood glucose level is met through hourly/twice-hourly bedside glucose monitoring.
- Once the target is met check again 1–2 hours later because sometimes the target range can be overshot.
- Once the patient is eating again, they can return to their previous regimen, utilizing the rapid-acting insulin correction to adjust for blood glucose over the target range.

Transition from an insulin infusion
It is important to remember the basic classification of AHAs and, more importantly, the contraindications for each of them (Table 10.1). Combination therapy that utilizes AHAs and/or insulin is a very useful diabetes regimen for those with T2 diabetes. **This regimen can be initiated in hospital; however, it should be noted that reassessment and adjustment will require outpatient follow-up.**

When returning to the previous AHA regimen, it is important to remember some basic pharmacokinetics. There will be some delay in the action of AHAs in lowering blood glucose levels once they have been started. So some overlap with insulin is best, i.e., the insulin infusion should continue until AHAs have begun to work (a few hours after the first dose). Alternatively, the insulin infusion could be stopped at the same time the AHA is started and the rapid-acting insulin CF could be used to maintain target blood glucose levels until the AHA has taken effect. It is logical (and safer) to begin the change in the regimen first thing in the morning to coincide with breakfast service and to allow assessment during the day when more ward staff is available.

When returning to the previous insulin regimen, the same approach applies. Remember to start with 15%—20% less of the "home dosage" to protect against hypoglycemia. The rapid-acting insulin CF will both maintain target blood glucose levels and provide a gauge for adjusting the total daily dose (TDD). The CF, along with the ordered rapid-acting premeal insulin, will help maintain target blood glucose levels until the basal insulin is given at the usual bedtime. Sometimes, particularly in people with T1 diabetes, it may be best to give ~25% of the basal insulin dose in the morning when transitioning, in order to prevent any possible development of ketones during the day.

When transitioning to a new insulin regimen, the 24-hour insulin requirements can be determined from the infusion and used as the "ballpark" starting TDD. The TDD can be distributed as best fits the situation. The approach currently being used is a basal/bolus insulin regimen. Basal insulin refers to either intermediate-acting (NPH) or long-acting (glargine, detemir, or degludec) insulin given as the "background" insulin od or bid. Bolus insulin refers to rapid-acting (lispro, aspart, or glulisine) insulin given with meals. Generally, 50% of the TDD is basal and 50% of the TDD is distributed as bolus. Further use of the rapid-acting insulin CF will provide the feedback for dosage adjustments. Remember, in individuals with T1 diabetes, it may be best to give ~25% of the basal insulin dose in the morning when transitioning, in order to prevent any possible development of ketones during the day.

Remember, a hospital is not the venue to establish a stable insulin dosage, as there are too many variables. The logical approach is to adjust the insulin dosage to maintain the safe target blood glucose range (5.0/6.0—10.0/12.0 mmol/L). **Detailed dosage adjustment is best done through postdischarge follow-up with a diabetes healthcare team.**

Key points for the medical ward
- Set a safe target blood glucose range, 5.0/6.0—10.0/12.0 mmol/L, that will be appropriate for most patients.

- Establish a starting diabetes regimen, whether AHA and/or insulin. Base it on the home regimen. In more stable patients, the TDD will be reduced by 15%–20% for safety to start. In less stable patients, the blood glucose levels may be higher; in this case the TDD will be increased by 10%–15% to start.
- Remember, it is always safer to titrate medication to adjust for higher blood glucose levels than to make a patient hypoglycemic.
- Avoid insulin sliding scales and avoid bolus insulin dosages in response to high blood glucose levels.
- For stable patients, use the rapid-acting insulin CF at mealtimes in addition to the set diabetes regimen.
- For more acutely ill patients who are not eating use either an insulin infusion or the rapid-acting insulin CF every 4–6 hours.

Special considerations

Any guide to diabetes management on the hospital ward would not be complete without specific mention of corticosteroids. Whether given orally, parenterally, in pulse or regular dosage regimens, steroids elevate blood glucose levels tremendously. Only aggressive use of insulin can address these elevations. In the person with known diabetes, aggressive augmentation of the pre-existing insulin regimen is required. Steroid use may "uncover" a diabetes predisposition and result in secondary diabetes. These people will need insulin de novo, as AHAs will rarely be sufficient.

The most common corticosteroid regimen is daily prednisone in the morning. This results in a pattern whereby blood glucose levels rise continuously throughout the day, then drop considerably overnight. Therefore insulin usually needs to be given in a large dose, i.e., rapid-acting and/or intermediate-/long-acting in a sufficiently high dose in the morning and a much lower dose in the evening.

Case study
Raymond

Raymond is a 61-year-old man admitted to hospital with a non-ST elevation myocardial infarction (NSTEMI). He is found to have new-onset T2 diabetes, with a random blood glucose of 20 mmol/L at the time of admission. He is being kept NPO pending a coronary angiography, with IV dextrose 50 cc/hour running.

The primary objective is to achieve and maintain a safe target blood glucose range of 5.0/6.0–10.0/12.0 mmol/L. With this degree of hyperglycemia and no set time for his procedure, the logical approach is to start an insulin infusion until he undergoes his angiography and he starts eating. If there is a set time for his procedure within the next 24 hours, then use of the rapid-acting insulin CF at "mealtimes" or every 4–6 hours can be used instead. Once he is able to eat, he can be transitioned to either continuing with a basal/bolus insulin regimen or a combination of AHAs and basal insulin.

Case study
Gwen

Gwen is a 50-year-old woman who is newly diagnosed with lymphoma and will be starting chemotherapy in hospital. High-dose corticosteroids are part of her chemotherapy protocol. She has T2 diabetes, which was previously controlled with gliclazide MR 60 mg od. After day 1 of her chemotherapy, her blood glucose level is 25 mmol/L, checked midafternoon.

The primary concern here is that high blood glucose levels will increase her risk of infection, along with the expected low white blood cell count she will experience from the chemotherapy. The sustained elevated blood glucose levels secondary to corticosteroids will respond only to insulin. There may be a pattern to the blood glucose levels. If the steroid is given once daily in the morning, the effect on blood glucose levels will be seen through the day and will taper off over 12 hours.

Accordingly, a logical approach is to give a combination of rapid-acting and basal (long-acting) insulin in the morning to provide continuous insulin coverage throughout the day. Set dosages of rapid-acting insulin and/or CF may be needed later in the day at mealtimes to bolster the sustained effect of the basal insulin.

Case study
Richard

Richard is a 73-year-old man with longstanding T2 diabetes for which he takes metformin 1000 mg bid, gliclazide MR 60 bid, and glargine insulin 20 units hs. He is admitted to hospital with pneumonia and dehydration. His serum creatinine level is rising as is his blood glucose level, which is currently 18 mmol/L.

The issue with Richard is not just maintaining a target blood glucose level; rather, the rising serum creatinine level and impending renal failure are of primary concern. Metformin should be decreased by 50% once the glomerular filtration rate reaches 60 mL/min and stopped once it reaches 30 mL/min. Clearance of other medications will also be affected, so the dosage of gliclazide will also need to be reduced.

The logical approach here would be to check his serum eGFR and either decrease or stop metformin depending on the value. There may be a need to increase the gliclazide if blood sugars rise once metformin is decreased or stopped. If he is not eating, then consideration should be given to decreasing his bedtime glargine dose by ~50% and using a mealtime CF of rapid-acting insulin during the day to maintain target blood sugars, or perhaps using an insulin infusion.

Once he recovers and his renal function returns to his baseline, it is very possible that his preadmission metformin dose can be reinstituted.

Diabetes on the surgical ward

All information regarding the medical ward also applies to the surgical ward. Here, however, the differences lie in a likely increased need for insulin infusions to carry the patients through the perioperative period when they are not eating. Maintaining target blood glucose levels is key to reduce the risk of perioperative sepsis. Therefore rapid-acting insulin CF can be very useful.

One major consideration on surgical wards is the common use of nutritional support, through either TF or TPN. The basic component of these two nutritional supports is glucose. Accordingly, blood glucose levels remain high in these patients. The only way to maintain target blood glucose levels is through the aggressive use of insulin. An insulin infusion is the most effective route.

The challenge comes when a TF regimen (less often, TPN) is changed from 24 hours to a modified time frame, in order to encourage oral feeding. Those modifications, such as overnight feeds or bolus feeds throughout the day, usually respond best to the use of rapid-acting insulin boluses, with the feeds supplemented by intermediate-/long-acting insulin od or bid.

A practical approach to blood glucose control in the surgical ward

For stable, less acutely ill patients utilize the patient's usual diabetes regimen with dosage adjustments as required. Some patients will need an increase in their dosage of ~10%—15% to accommodate the initial stress of hospitalization. But remember, once that initial situation has stabilized, there will likely be a need to reduce dosage by at least 15%—20% to account for the strictly controlled hospital diet.

Use the rapid-acting insulin CF at mealtimes to maintain the target blood glucose range as follows: give 1—2 units for every 3.0 mmol/L greater than 12 mmol/L (the upper target range). This CF can be used alongside any existing diabetes regimen.

Acutely ill patients who are unable or not allowed to eat and perioperative patients who are still not eating are best controlled by an insulin infusion:

- Start with regular/rapid-acting insulin at 1 unit/hour IV simultaneously running with D5W at 50—75 cc/hour. The D5W provides some CHO substrate for the insulin.
- Titrate the insulin infusion ± 1 unit/hour at a time until the target blood glucose level is met through hourly/twice-hourly bedside glucose monitoring.
- Once target is met check again 1—2 hours later, as sometimes the target range can be overshot.
- Once the patient is eating again, the patient can be transferred back to the previous regimen, utilizing the rapid-acting insulin correction algorithm to adjust for blood glucose level over the target range.

Key points

1. Set a safe target blood glucose range: 5.0/6.0—10.0/12.0 mmol/L will be appropriate for most patients.
2. Establish a regular diabetes regimen, whether AHA and/or insulin, that is based upon the home regimen. In more stable patients, the TDD should be reduced by 15%—20% for safety to start. In less stable patients, whose blood glucose levels may be higher, the TDD should be increased by 15%—20% to start.
3. Avoid insulin sliding scales and bolus insulin dosages in response to high blood glucose levels.
4. Use the rapid-acting insulin CF at mealtimes instead, in addition to the set diabetes regimen.

5. For acutely ill patients, or those patients who are postoperative and not yet eating, use either the rapid-acting insulin CF every 4–6 hours or an insulin infusion. Once they are able to eat transfer them back to their previous diabetes regimen.
6. Remember, TF and TPN are significant sources of glucose. Insulin, in higher dosages will be required to maintain adequate control, generally by insulin infusion.

Case study
Stan

Stan is a 55-year-old man with longstanding T2 diabetes for which he takes gliclazide MR 60 mg od. He has been admitted to hospital with an infected diabetic foot ulcer. He requires a number of surgical debridement procedures in the operating room, as well as an aortogram to assess the possibility of an aortofemoral bypass. Currently, he is NPO on standby. His blood glucose level is 18.0 mmol/L.

The issue here is maintaining the target blood glucose level of 5.0/6.0–12.0 mmol/L while he is on standby throughout the day. The logical approach is to start an insulin infusion.

Then, as often happens, Stan is bumped from the emergency slate and allowed to eat, but he will be NPO after midnight on standby for the operating room tomorrow.

The logical approach is to still use insulin. There are two options:

1. *Insulin administration could be stopped but he would need a rapid-acting insulin dose for supper. This dose could be calculated as an extrapolation from his hourly requirements throughout the day, such as if he is requiring 2 units/hour, 48 units/day. This calculation results in 24 units basal and 24 units divided among the three meals or 8 units for a meal. Adding the CF at meals will help maintain target blood glucose level. As he will be NPO after midnight, he probably needs only 15%–25% of the calculated basal dose at bedtime.*
2. *He could continue with the insulin infusion utilizing a square-wave bolus for his supper (i.e., increase the insulin infusion rate by 2 units for 2 hours over the mealtime).*

Discharge planning

Utilizing the strategies elucidated in this chapter, blood glucose levels can usually be maintained in the hospital. The potential for problems occurs after discharge. Deterioration of blood glucose control can happen quite easily once a patient is home. Usually, hyperglycemia occurs related to a combination of inactivity and a change in nutritional intake. Hyperglycemia increases the risk of sepsis and introduces the real possibility of readmission to hospital. This risk applies to medical and surgical patients alike; however, the risk may be greater for the surgical patient with a healing incision. Follow-up assessment in a timely fashion can reduce this risk.

The need to arrange postdischarge assessment cannot be overstated. This assessment may occur in a variety of ways: through a primary care provider, a hospital or community-based diabetes healthcare team, and/or a designated diabetes case manager. The key is to provide support to adjust AHAs and/or insulin dosages to maintain the target blood glucose range. While the optimal target blood glucose range is 4.0–7.0 mmol/L premeal and 5.0–8.0 mmol/L 2 hours postmeal (10.0 mmol/L for those susceptible to hypoglycemia), these targets may vary depending on the situation. Postdischarge blood glucose control should be tighter for those recovering from surgery and/or sepsis to decrease any further risk of sepsis.

Newly diagnosed individuals will require basic diabetes survival skills before leaving hospital, including self-monitoring of blood glucose levels, insulin administration, and recognition and treatment of hypoglycemia. Most importantly, they need to be connected to community-based follow-up for their diabetes.

APPENDIX 1

Unit conversion table: mmol/L to mg/dL

mmol/L	Conversion factor to mg/dL
Apolipoprotein B	× 100
β-hydroxybutyrate	÷ 104.1
Blood glucose	× 18
Cholesterol	× 38.67
Creatinine	× 0.0113
High-density lipoprotein cholesterol	× 38.67
Low-density lipoprotein cholesterol	× 38.67
Non-high-density lipoprotein cholesterol	× 38.67
Triglycerides	× 88.57

INDEX

Note: Page numbers followed by *"f"* indicate figures and *"t"* indicate tables.

Printed in the United States
by Baker & Taylor Publisher Services